Contents

KU-060-640

0•4 Author's acknowledgements

The health of men and the health of women are often inextricably linked. Prostate cancer makes a lot of women very ill. Similarly, cervical cancer makes a lot of men very ill. Chlamydia is not an edible shell fish. It is the single greatest cause of female infertility, pelvic inflammatory disease and ectopic pregnancy. In men it generally only causes an itchy willy. It takes two to tango and improving men's insight into women's health may actually have a positive effect on their own health.

This manual was also a partnership effort. Jim Campbell interpreted the message faultlessly and brought lipsticks to life while Suzie Hayman gave them insight and common sense. Matthew Minter provided the orchestra for the dance but insider information scores best every time. Hilary Martelli gave a second opinion only possible from someone deficient in Y chromosomes. Simon Gregory cast a technical eye over the manuscript and Ian Barnes imposed order on what looked suspiciously like chaos.

The similarity between sections of the manual and the NHS Direct health guide and encyclopaedia is no coincidence and we give thankful acknowledgment to Bob Gann and his team at NHS Direct On Line.

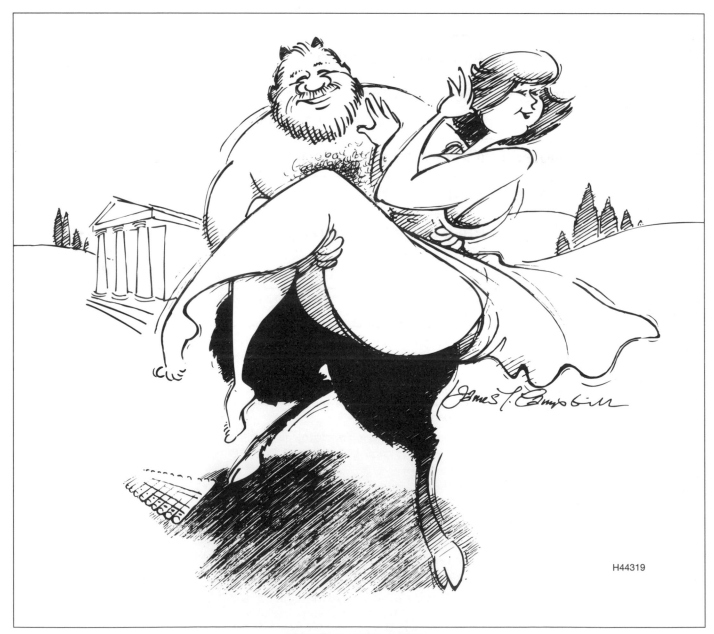

H44319

The author and his goddess

Write down the symptoms before you see the doctor

• It is easy to forget the most important things during the examination. Doctors home-in on important clues. When did it start? How did it feel? Did anyone else suffer as well? Did this ever happen before? Has anything been done about it so far? Is the sufferer on any medicines at present?

Arrive informed

• Check out the net for information before going to the surgery. There are thousands of sites on health but many of them are of little real use. Click on the NHS Direct On Line or female health sites for up to date accurate and unbiased information.

Ask questions

• If a mechanic stuck his head under the bonnet of a car you would most certainly want to know what he intended doing. This doctor is about to lift the bonnet...

Watch out for over investigation

• Litigation against doctors is now big business. Defensive medicine can lead to unnecessary tests and investigations. Most X-ray examinations of the painful low-back are completely useless. Similarly, isolated cholesterol tests can be misleading. Ask whether the test will really help diagnosis and treatment.

Avoid asking for night visits unless there is a good reason

• Calling a GP after 'suffering' all day at work will antagonise a doctor who thinks personal health should come before convenience. If money is put before the quality of family life don't be surprised if asked to come to the surgery the following morning.

Don't prevaricate

• If there is a lump, say so. There are thousands cases of breast cancer each year in the UK. With an average of only seven minutes for each consultation there is a real danger of coming out with a prescription for a sore nose.

Health promotion as once decreed by the government is no more

• Now is the time to convince the family doctor to take a serious look at health. Little screening system exists at present but nothing prevents you from asking for a consultation to examine risk factors. A strong family history of conditions such as heart disease, diabetes, cancer or eye problems like glaucoma should prompt some basic tests.

Listen to what the doctor says

• It helps if they write down the important points. Most people pick up less than half of what their doctor has told them.

Have your prescription explained

• Three items on a scrip will cost you as much as a half decent tyre. Ask whether they can be bought across the counter. What are they all for? Some medicines clash badly with alcohol. Even one pint of beer with the popular antibiotic metronidazole (Flagyl) will make you feel very ill. Mixing antidepressants and alcohol can be fatal. Are there any side effects you should look out for?

If you want a second opinion say so

• Ask for a consultant appointment by all means but remember you are dealing with a person with feelings and not a computer. Compliment him for his attention first but then explain your deep anxiety.

Flattery will get you anywhere

• Praise is thin on the ground these days. An acknowledgment of a good effort, even if not successful, will be remembered.

Be consistent with all the staff

• Receptionists are not all dragons and practice nurses increasingly influence your treatment. General practice is a team effort and you will get the best out of it by treating all its members with respect.

Be prepared to complain

• If possible see the doctor first and explain what is annoying you. Most complaints against doctors are for rudeness and poor communication, usually as a result of work pressure. Family doctors now have an 'in-house' complaints system. If still not satisfied you can take it to a formal hearing.

Trust your doctor

• There is a difference between trust and blind faith. Your health is a partnership between you and your doctor where you are the majority stakeholder. Despite everything successive governments have done to the NHS the majority of people who work in it are still driven by vocation.

Change your GP with caution

• Thousands of people change their doctor each year. Most of them have simply moved house. You do not need to tell your family doctor if you wish to leave their practice. Your new doctor will arrange for all your notes to be transferred. The whole point of general practice is to build up a personal insight into the health of you and your family. A new doctor has to start almost from scratch.

Don't be afraid to ask to see your notes

• Most doctors now show their patients what they are writing. Unfortunately doctors' language can be difficult to understand. Latin and Greek are still in use although on the decline. Doctors use abbreviations in your notes. Watch out for:

a) *SUPRATENTORIAL: Conscious thought and automatic bodily functions are located in different parts of the brain separated by a membrane called the tentorium. The upper part looks after personality, memory, writing and speech. Below the tentorium the brain makes sure you are still breathing. If your doctor thinks you are deluding yourself over your symptoms the real problem lies above the tentorium.*

b) *HYSTERIA: A dangerous diagnosis. Few doctors will be brave (or stupid) enough to write this in their notes.*

c) *TATT: An abbreviation for Tired All The Time.*

d) *TCA SOS: To Call Again if things get worse. Most illnesses are self-limiting. A couple of weeks usually allows nature to sort things out.*

e) *RV: Review. Secretaries will automatically arrange a subsequent appointment.*

f) *PEARLA: Pupils Equal and Reacting to Light and Accommodation. A standard entry on a casualty sheet to show that your brain is functioning.*

g) *C_2H_5OH: The chemical formula for ethyl alcohol.*

h) *RTA: Road Traffic Accident.*

i) *FROM: Full Range Of Movement at a joint.*

j) *SOB: Short Of Breath. If this comes on after walking in from the waiting room it turns into SOBOE – On Exercise.*

k) *AMA/CMA: Against Medical Advice/Contrary Medical Advice: You went home despite medical advice not to do so.*

l) *DNA: Did Not Attend. You didn't turn up for your appointment.*

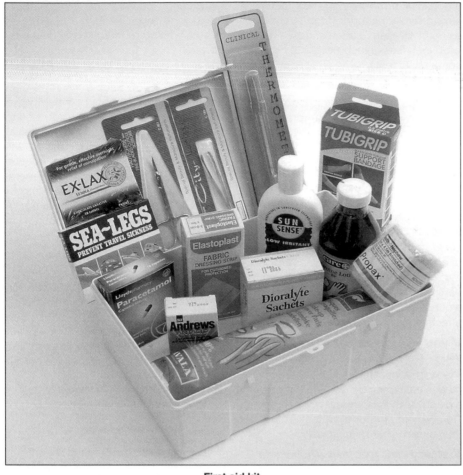

First aid kit

Minor illnesses or accidents can happen at any time so it's worth being prepared. It makes sense to keep some first aid and simple remedies in a safe place in the house to cover most minor ailments and accidents.

- Painkillers.
- Mild laxatives.
- Anti-diarrhoeal, rehydration mixture.
- Indigestion remedy, eg, antacids.
- Travel sickness tablets.
- Sunscreen – SPF30 or higher.
- Sunburn treatment.
- Tweezers, sharp scissors.
- Thermometer.
- A selection of plasters, cotton wool, elastic bandages and assorted dressings.

Remember

- Keep the medicine chest in a secure, locked place, out of reach of small children.
- Do not keep in the bathroom as the damp will soon damage the medicines and bandages.
- Always read the instructions and use the right dose.
- Watch expiry dates – don't keep or use medicines past their sell-by date.

lipstick

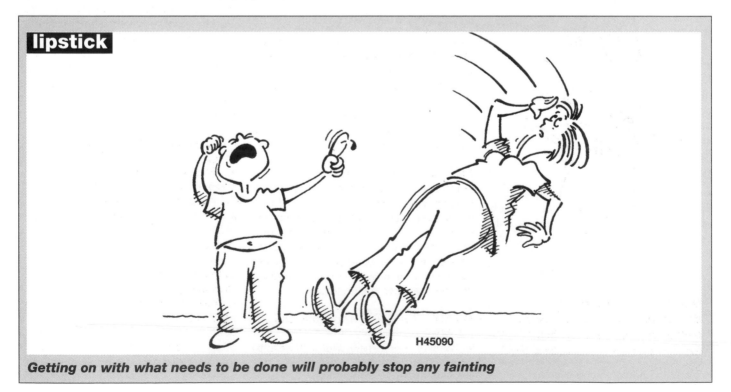

Getting on with what needs to be done will probably stop any fainting

Chapter 1
Roadside repairs (first aid)

Contents

1 First aid

Accidents account for greatest loss of life amongst the young. Car crashes, sports injuries, industrial accidents and dodgy DIY are all major causes of injury and death.

Having someone around with first aid knowledge can make the difference. Anyone can learn these simple but often life saving techniques.

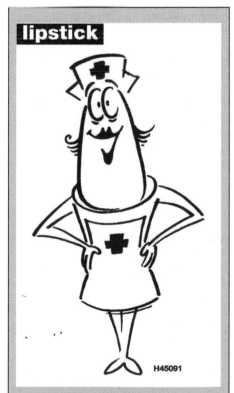

If a little knowledge is dangerous then perhaps we'd better make sure we have lots – I vote we enrol in a first aid course!

2 Myths of first aid

Below are some commonly asked questions and answers:

You will be successfully sued if you look after someone and they think you were negligent:
• **Wrong:** The good Samaritan principle should keep you safe from successful litigation in most cases. You are only expected to be able to do what any other non-medically trained person could do.

Men should not look after injured women in case they are accused of sexual harassment:
• **Wrong:** Common-sense prevails. Do what you need to do to save her life. If another woman is present, use her to chaperone. Explain out loud what you are doing even if she appears unconscious, it also helps to calm onlookers.

People always faint when they see all the blood:
• **Wrong.** If you know what you need to do and you get on with it you will probably not faint.

You will catch HIV if you perform mouth to mouth resuscitation on someone with AIDS:
• **Wrong:** Although there is a small theoretical risk, the chances of becoming infected are extremely small.

First aid makes no difference. Getting them to hospital takes precedence:
• **Wrong:** It is vital to get professional help as soon as possible but ambulance drivers generally like to pick up live people on the way to casualty. A person can lose all their blood from a serious wound in a relatively short space of time. You can save someone's life before the ambulance even arrives. After one hour, the so called 'Golden Hour', a person's fate is more or less sealed. You make the difference in the equation.

A little knowledge is a dangerous thing:
• **Wrong:** This is usually quoted by people who would rather not bother. So long as you stick to what you know and use common sense it is unlikely you will make the situation any worse.

Doing something is always better than doing nothing:
• **Wrong.** People with no idea can be a danger to your health. Giving a badly injured person alcohol might bring their colour back but if they're bleeding it could kill them. Get trained.

1

3 It seemed like a good idea (common mistakes)

We all carry ideas on what to do in an emergency. Most of them come from the movies.

Don't give a casualty anything to eat or drink.

• If a person is unable to swallow properly, for example after a stroke or head injury, you could choke them, and if they need surgery the anaesthetist would not thank you.

Don't leave an unconscious or drunk person lying on their back.

• Vomit or even their own tongue could block their airway. Stay with them, but shout to attract help or if possible use a mobile telephone.

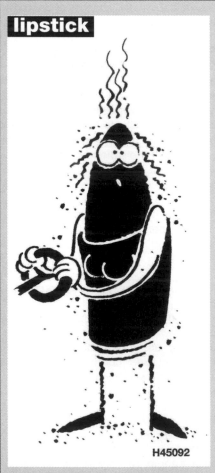

First thing to do in a car crash? Check the ignition is turned off!

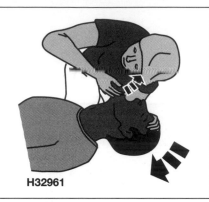

4.5 Clear the airway by extending the head backwards

Don't be afraid to call the emergency services.

• If you are not sure whether you are out of your depth you probably are. Send two people to phone at the same time. Get one to return and let you know what's happening, and tell one to stay and direct the ambulance.

Don't use a tourniquet.

• Once a tourniquet is released all the debris in the blood blocks up the kidneys. Instead press firmly on the wound to stop the bleeding.

Don't put yourself in danger.

• If it goes wrong the emergency services have two casualties to deal with. Check your surroundings first for falling rocks, fumes, cars, live electricity, etc.

4 Cardio-pulmonary resuscitation (kiss of life)

Simply reading how to perform cardio-pulmonary-resuscitation (CPR) is like expecting to be able to drive a Porsche after reading the workshop manual. You need to be trained before having to do it for real.

1 Take a moment to check you are not in danger. Look around and make sure you will be safe to help.

2 Try and get the person to respond, talk to them, gently squeeze their shoulder. Look for even small movements and listen carefully. If you get no response shout for help. Dial 999/112 from a mobile or landline.

3 Check the ABC (that's Airway, Breathing and Circulation):

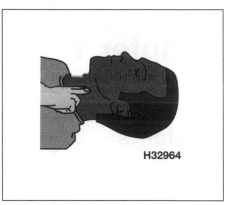

4.8 Checking for a pulse at the artery in the neck

4 First clear the airway (A). Tip the head backwards extremely gently, and clear anything out of the mouth.

5 Listen carefully for breathing (B). Look along the chest for movement and place your ear and cheek close to the injured person's mouth to listen and feel for breathing.

6 If the patient is not breathing then start the first part of CPR (cardio-pulmonary resuscitation), the so-called Kiss of Life.

7 Pinch the person's nose, take a deep breath and then place your lips over the person's mouth, trying to create a seal. Then steadily blow over a period of two seconds (this is one 'ventilation'). Watch to see the chest wall rise. If there is no movement then readjust the airway and try again. You can attempt this five times. Once it works make sure you get two full breaths in.

8 Now you need to check the patient's circulation (C). Check for a pulse (using your first two fingers) at the artery in the neck, found on the left side of the neck, just under the chin. Take up to 10 seconds to check this properly, and look at the person's colour, temperature and generally any signs of life.

9 If there is no signs of circulation perform the second part of CPR, chest compressions or heart massage.

10 First locate the right hand position. Put your middle finger at the point where the bottom ribs meet the sternum (chest bone). Place your index finger above it and then place the heel of your other hand next to it. Using both hands together compress the chest straight down to a third of its depth.

11 Compress the chest 15 times quite

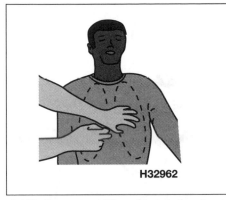

4.10A Correct position of hands for chest compressions

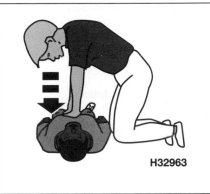

4.10B Keep arms straight with each thrust

quickly (a rate of 100 compressions per minute), followed by two ventilations. Continue CPR like this until:
• Emergency help arrives or another rescuer offers assistance.
• The patient shows signs of life. Reassess breathing and circulation.
• You become exhausted and cannot continue.
• It becomes unsafe.

5 Broken bones

Bones contain blood vessels and nerves. A fracture is painful, more so if the broken ends are sticking into flesh. Follow these simple rules:
1 Tell the injured person to keep still. Steady and support the limb with your hands.
2 Cover any wounds with a dressing or clean non fluffy material, eg shirt. Press as hard as required to stop the bleeding. Bandage the dressing onto the limb.
3 If a leg is broken, tie both legs together with a piece of wood or rolled up magazines between them. Tie the knees and ankles together first then closer to the broken bone.
4 Suspected broken arms or collar bones should be supported by fastening the arm on the affected side to the body.
5 Always check that the hands or feet are warm and colour returns after squeezing a nail. If not, loosen the bandages a little.
6 Swelling can tighten bandages so check every fifteen minutes.

6 Broken spine

A broken neck or spine will not necessarily kill or paralyse you, but if you suspect a broken spine it is essential you follow these simple rules.
1 Do not move the person unless there is imminent danger within the area. If they must be moved, always support the head on each side with gentle but firm pulling and use a number of people to lift in as many places as possible. If possible use a flat piece of wood to carry them while still supporting their head.
2 Reassure the person and tell them not to move. Steady the head with hands on either side of the ears.
3 Get helpers to place rolled blankets or coats around the sides to stop them rolling.
4 Dial 999 or 112 and explain what has happened.
5 Continue to check their breathing while you wait for help.

7 Dislocated joints

Dislocating any joint can damage surrounding nerves, blood vessels, and ligaments. Trying to force the joint back into place can make this ten times worse. Dislocated shoulders are common because it is a relatively lax joint. Horrendous damage can be done by well meaning offers to 'pop it back in'.

1 Simply support the arm against the front of the body and get the patient to casualty. Don't give them anything to eat or drink as they may need a general anaesthetic.

8 Burns

1 Cool the burn area with cold water. This can take 10 minutes. Send someone for the ambulance if the burn is severe (greater in size than the size of their own palm).
2 Remove watches, bracelets or anything which will cause constriction once the flesh begins to swell. This includes shoes and necklaces.
3 **Don't** remove clothes if they are sticking to the skin.
4 Cover the burn area with light non-fluffy material.
5 Don't apply creams or burst any blisters.
6 With severe burns there will be a rapid loss of fluid from the blood system with a loss of blood pressure. Lay them down and raise their legs. This helps keep blood available for the vital organs as well as the heart, brain, kidney and lungs.

9 Choking

It takes surprisingly little to choke a person. Here's what to do if you see someone choking:
1 Check inside their mouth. If you can see the offending obstruction pull it out. If you can't see it, bend the patient over and use the flat of your hand to slap them firmly on the back between the shoulder blades five times.
2 If all this fails, go for the Heimlich manoeuvre (the abdominal thrust).
3 Stand behind the person. Put both arms around the waist and interlock your hands.
4 Pull sharply upwards below the ribs. Try five times and go back to number one.

1

10 Eye injury

Eyes are amazingly tough. Blows from blunt instruments, such as a squash ball, cause extensive damage to the surrounding bone but the eye usually remains intact. Penetrating injuries are a different matter. Flakes of steel from a chisel struck with a hammer travel at the speed of sound. That's significantly faster than the blink of an eye.

1 Lay the patient on their back and examine the eye. Only wash the eye if there is no obvious foreign body stuck to the eye and it has no open wound.

2 Place a loose pad over the eye and bandage.

3 Take them to hospital.

11 Heart attacks

Heart disease is the single biggest killer of women so you are likely to see it happen at some time. Modern treatment can significantly improve chances of survival if you can get her to hospital quickly. Recognise what's going on. Central chest pain can move upwards to the throat or arms, usually the left arm.

1 Fear causes the release of adrenaline which makes the heart beat faster, increasing the pain, so talk calmly and reassure.

2 Call for an ambulance.

3 If they normally take a tablet or oral spray for chest pain, let them do so. Give them an aspirin to chew on, it stops any more clot forming in their coronary blood vessels which caused the heart attack. Don't give them anything else to eat or drink.

4 Sit them down but don't force them to lie down if they don't want to.

5 If you would like to know more, look in the Contacts section at the back of this manual, or contact:

British Heart Foundation
14 Fitzhardinge Street, London W1H 6DH
020 7935 0185
www.bhf.org.uk.

12 Heavy bleeding

1 Lay them down. Bleeding from a vein is generally slow and simply pressing a cloth against the wound and raising the affected limb above the level of the heart will stop the bleeding. Get them to hospital.

2 Arterial bleeds can be seriously different. It's hard to miss when it happens. The blood is bright red and comes out in spurts with each heart beat.

3 Press a cloth against the wound and hold it down firmly. If you have to leave them, secure it to the wound with a shirt or towel.

4 Raise their arms and legs to keep the blood pressure up. Some seepage will occur but you may save their life. Get them to hospital.

13 Do the knowledge

The principles of First Aid are easy when explained by an expert on a training course. Whether you end up reassuring an elderly relative after a fall, or saving a choking child, the sense of reward is amazing. The following charities offer courses, why not give them a call today:

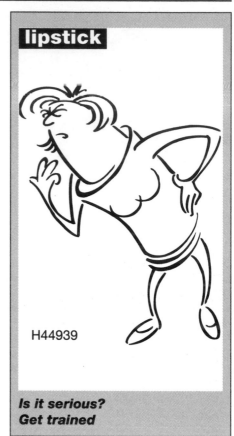

lipstick

H44939

Is it serious?
Get trained

British Heart Foundation,
14 Fitzhardinge Street,
London,
W1H 6DH.
020 7935 0185
www.bhf.org.uk

St John Ambulance,
27 St. John's Lane,
London,
EC1M 4BU.
0870-010 4950
www.sja.org.uk

Chapter 2
Bodywork and chassis (skin and bones)

Contents

1   Athlete's foot

1   Fungus just loves damp dark places to grow in, so areas of broken skin especially between the toes are a sure sign of Tinea, also responsible for so called 'ringworm' elsewhere on the skin. Its ability to infect other people has been overstated in the past.

Symptoms

• Raw, itchy broken skin between the toes which looks white and boggy when damp.

• Wearing trainers for a while soon produces a strong smell.

• Bending toes can be painful; they can also be tender to the touch or while wearing shoes.

Causes

• The fungus can be picked up from swimming pools, baths or even wet floors.

• Sharing towels or footwear can transfer the fungus between people.

• Wearing trainers without socks makes it easier for infection to take hold.

Prevention

• Dry and well-ventilated feet rarely become infected with fungus.

• Drying them after each wash, twice per day is essential, especially between the toes.

• Talcum powder is made from chalk and fish scales. It only makes things worse.

• Wool or cotton socks are better than man-made fibres.

• Footwear, especially trainers, should have plenty of ventilation.

• Walking around the house barefoot really helps and also stops calluses forming.

• Wearing trainers without socks is tempting fate (feet?).

Complications

2   Skin loss can be severe with

2

secondary infection from bacteria. This can be very dangerous in people who are diabetic.

3 The infection can spread into the nails causing disfigurement and discolouration. The nails can become incredibly thick which can be painful as well as unsightly.

Self care

4 Keeping feet dry for an extended period can help but often an antifungal cream or powder will be needed to clear up the infection completely.

5 Antifungal creams and powders can now be bought across the counter without prescription but must be used continuously until after a couple of weeks of fungus-free feet.

6 Toe nail infections require prolonged courses (around 4-6 weeks) of antifungal drugs available only through prescription.

2 Boils

1 Historical treatment of boils verges on torture. Victorian England was obsessed with them as an obvious sign of poor hygiene and bad living. Boils generally form from infected hair follicles. If this is on the eye lid it is called a stye. Staphylococcus bacteria are the commonest cause and the body reacts to it by building a wall around it. Unfortunately this also impedes the body's natural defences from attacking the bacteria and a cyst, or boil, develops. After a certain length of time the skin lying over the boil will break down releasing the pus. Carbuncles are just collections of boils very close together and are thankfully not seen very often.

Symptoms

2 It's hard to miss a boil. A painful red lump appears on the skin which gradually gets larger and more painful. The area around the boil is also very tender and slightly inflamed. After a few days a white/yellow 'head' forms which means the boil is about to burst through the skin to release the pus and ease the pain. Some boils will disappear without actually releasing the pus through the skin.

Causes

3 Being 'run down' or suffering from some illness which lowers the body's defence against infection can increase your risk from boils. 'Dirty' skin is not a cause of boils. Over washing with antiseptic soaps may even increase your risk. Generally we don't know why some people develop boils more than others but the back of the neck is a common site.

Prevention

4 There is no real prevention against boils but persistent boils should be reported to a doctor.

Complications

5 Some boils can persist and come back again in the same place. This may leave a scar.

Self care

6 Once the head has formed the boil can be made to break by using warm water compresses. Soak some cotton wool in warm water mixed with a couple of spoonfuls of salt. Press it against the boil gently squeezing at the same time. Do not use the highly dangerous method of putting the mouth of a heated bottle to the boil then cooling the bottle to 'draw' the pus. It can cause infection into the blood stream and may leave a scar. Styes are best left alone as they burst after a short time. If they persist or are very painful they can be encouraged to disappear by gently dabbing with a clean

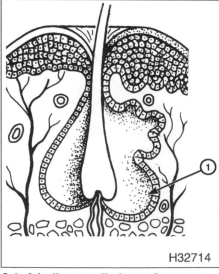

2.1 A boil generally forms from a pus-filled hair follicle (1)

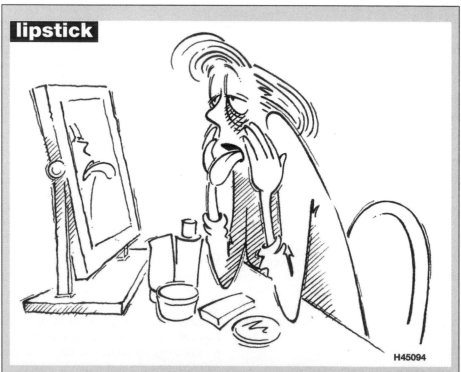

lipstick

H45094

Being 'run down' or suffering from some illness which lowers the body's defence against infection can increase your risk from boils

cloth damp with warm water. Do not attempt to open the stye.

More information

7 Persistent boils can occur if the body's defences against infection are affected by conditions such as diabetes or HIV. Long courses of steroids can also lower resistance to infection. Some doctors will prescribe antibiotics but others feel that this may delay the natural eruption of the boil through the skin. Once the head is formed some doctors will lance the boil by cutting into the head and breaking down all the layers within the boil allowing it to drain freely.

8 Staphylococcus also causes a particularly nasty food poisoning which comes on quite soon after eating infected food. Handling food at home requires certain precautions:

• Cover the boil.
• Wash hands frequently.
• Make sure there is no contact with food.

9 Working in any capacity with the preparation or serving of food for public consumption is not allowed if there is a danger of contamination from a boil.

3 Corns

1 Shoes have a lots to answer for, even the posh versions, as people who always walk barefoot do not develop corns. Localised skin thickening occurs over areas which are under constant pressure or rubbing, the sole of the foot is a normal and natural place for this but the backs of the toes can only develop thickening from shoe friction. Classically they will form over the back of the toes or where the toes join the foot. Corns will also form over the ball of the foot although walking barefoot regularly helps even out the skin. Calluses are also simply thick skin often seen on the hands of people doing heavy manual work.

Symptoms

2 Although thick skin itself is not painful it causes a pressure from the shoe on the soft parts of the foot underneath with

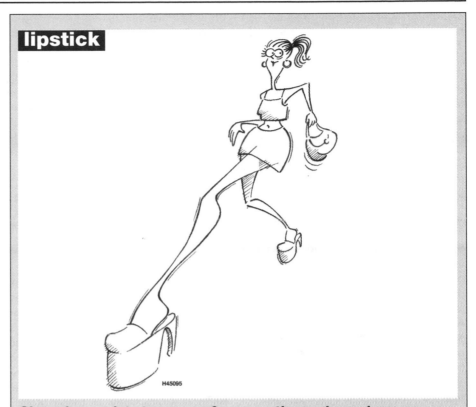

Shoes have a lots to answer for, even the posh versions, as people who always walk barefoot do not develop corns

bruising, pain and even bleeding with subsequent infection. Calluses on the hands reduce sensitivity – important for intimacy not to mention dexterity for handling small objects.

Causes

3 Although badly-fitting shoes are the commonest cause of corns they can form with good fitting shoes and excessive walking. The Chinese tradition of binding feet, now abandoned, caused dreadful corns and disfigurement. The modern equivalent is the high heel stiletto.

Prevention

4 Fashion dictates to a large extent but alternating fashionable footwear with barefoot walking will help. Even walking around the house or office barefoot can make a big difference.

Complications

5 It is rare for the corn to cause anything else other than pain and

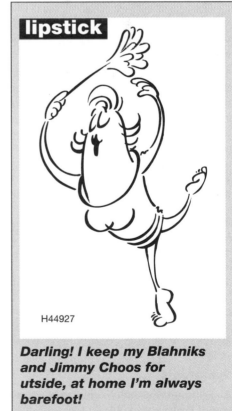

Darling! I keep my Blahniks and Jimmy Choos for utside, at home I'm always barefoot!

discomfort but constant bruising can cause a deep ulcer beneath the corn. These are notoriously difficult to treat once well developed so people with diabetes should beware of this as they may not feel the pain and allow the ulcer to grow and become infected. Regular foot care is essential and feet should be checked regularly by a chiropodist. Soothing as they are, hot foot spas should be avoided for the same reason as they can cause an infection. Keeping the feet dry is very important as bacteria thrive in moist warm places.

Self care

6 Changing to well-fitting shoes will make the corn disappear. Corn removal pastes and plasters from the pharmacist do work but the corn will reappear when continuing to wear badly-fitting shoes. Although pumice stones and sandpaper are also very effective to reduce the size of the corn, heavy handedness will cause bleeding and infection. Again, diabetic people must never do this for obvious reasons. Corn pads (soft rubber cushion pads) can reduce the friction but may actually increase the pressure, making things worse.

4 Cramp

1 There are very special times when cramp hits. It never happens when watching TV. Too simple, it always kicks in during love making when the slightest twitch of the little toe brings on agonising spasms of calf pain. A true test of any relationship. Hopping around the floor like a demented pogo stick demands a certain sense of humour on all sides. In truth few of us will never suffer cramp at some time. Muscle spasm which lasts for a few minutes most often occurs in the lower legs and feet. Lack of oxygen may be a factor but in most cases there appears to be no real reason although it happens more often while lying in bed. Unfortunately there are some serious conditions which will cause repeated attacks of cramp particularly when walking.

Symptoms

2 Although the body is kind enough to give a degree of warning, it is similar to the bomb disposal expert's dilemma of 'blue wire or green wire' when it comes to prevention. Such is the body's perverted sense of humour, cutting both wires will still result in demented pogo. There is a warning tightness of the muscle with a small degree of pain. Movement at this point seems to trigger a full blown attack and the muscle tightens into a hard ball over which there is no control. Indeed trying to move it only makes the pain and tightening worse. Eventually the pain and tightness subsides but here is a feeling that another movement would trigger a fresh attack.

Causes

3 Overtiredness, dehydration, overexertion, sitting for prolonged periods, for example, on a plane journey and overheating are all undisputed factors but exercising with a full stomach is also said to cause cramp. A common factor has to be poor blood supply to the muscles or overexertion, yet cramp can happen without any of these factors being present.

Prevention

4 Although athletes use warm up exercises before strenuous activity such as running or swimming which not only help avoid cramp, they also prevent tendon injury such as a ruptured Achilles, this is not quite the bedroom answer. Women often complain of cramp during the pre-menstrual period. Now is the time to offer a massage rather than a wham, blam cheerio Ma'am approach to cramp.

Complications

5 On Saturday afternoons A&E departments across the UK are full of young rugby players whose helpful front row prop offered to 'just pop' a dislocated shoulder back in place. Monday morning solicitors offices specialising in divorce are probably also filled with women whose helpful partner offered to cure her cramp by forcing her toe, foot or limb against the cramp. This can tear the muscle or its ligaments. The pain then lasts much longer particularly with movement and is often described by court plaintiffs as being 'hopping mad'.

Self care

6 Cramp will eventually disappear on its own but can be helped by gentle and empathic massage of the affected muscle and gradual movement of the limb, foot or toe without saying 'are you ready now'.

5 Dandruff

1 Flaky skin falling from the scalp is just as common in women and although psoriasis will cause dandruff, the commonest cause is seborrhoeic eczema. Both produce flaky white scales but the eczema tends to be slightly waxy and as women tend to wear their hair longer there is the added complication of too frequent washing and conditioning. At the end of the day, and it usually is, we spend an enormous amount as a society on something which is completely harmless.

Symptoms

2 Dandruff causes nothing other than white snow from above. There may be a slight itch although this is often caused by inflammation from scratching. White flakes of dead skin will fall from the scalp particularly when combing or brushing

Causes

3 Seborrhoeic eczema is poorly understood and may be as simple as a reaction to chemicals. There is an overproduction of skin which builds up around the bases of the hair follicles. There is usually no infective agent involved although Tinea (ringworm) will cause hair loss, itching and some dandruff (see *Ringworm*).

Prevention

4 Although there is no shortage of 'anti dandruff' shampoos on the market the truth is that over zealous washing with harsh soaps or detergents will often make things worse. Regular washing and brushing may help keep the dandruff at bay but paradoxically may stimulate it.

Complications

5 Lots of dandruff does not relate to lots of hair loss unless there is an infection such as Tinea (ringworm).

Self care

6 Anti dandruff shampoos do work although they need to used over a long period. Once they are stopped the dandruff often returns. Some of them are based on formaldehyde which is used to preserve tissue and specimens; overuse is inviting other problems such as scalp irritations. Similarly strong soaps and over use of hair gels should be avoided.

6 German Measles (Rubella)

1 This highly infectious condition is now uncommon thanks to the MMR vaccine.

Symptoms

2 The person is rarely ill but will have a mildly raised temperature and swollen glands on the neck and base of the skull. Pin-head sized flat, red spots last around two days and need no treatment other than some paracetamol for the slight fever.

Causes

3 The virus is very contagious and will spread quickly in a population lacking immunity.

Prevention

4 Vaccination for girls and boys is both safe and effective.

Complications

5 Very rarely the virus that causes German Measles (Rubella) will cause an inflammation of the brain (encephalitis).
6 The real danger may come in later life if an unvaccinated woman becomes infected with German Measles (Rubella) while pregnant. This can cause brain damage, deafness and other congenital problems for the unborn child. For these major reasons both boys and girls should be immunised with this very safe vaccine.

Self care

• Paracetamol will reduce the mild fever.

7 Hair loss

1 Hair is essentially dead except for the so-called roots, or follicles. This is a happy coincidence for hairdressers who would otherwise need to use a general anaesthetic every time they gave a perm. Hair loss is often a butt of other people's jokes but can be a major problem for women, undermining their self confidence. Many cultures favour cutting off a woman's hair for some perceived treachery.
2 Hair usually contains pigment but air bubbles give hair a silvery colour. The root of each hair is contained in a tubular pit of the skin called the hair follicle. A minute muscle, the erector pili, is attached to each hair follicle to make the hair 'stand on end'. Hair growth rate varies with age, person and with the hair length. Short hair grows at about 2 cm per month; by the time the hair is a foot long, the rate of growth is reduced by one-half. Young women's hair between 16 and 24 years grows fastest.

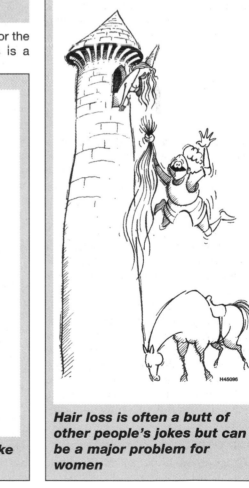

Hair loss is often a butt of other people's jokes but can be a major problem for women

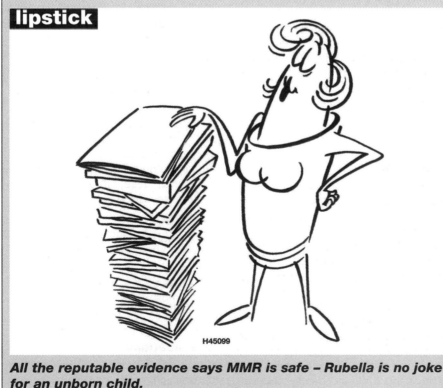

All the reputable evidence says MMR is safe – Rubella is no joke for an unborn child.

2

Causes of hair loss

• Age, although this does vary between women.

• Pregnancy stops the normal hair growth and loss cycle in its tracks. Soon after the baby is born the cycle is restored but generally in the hair loss phase.

• Ringworm infections cause localised hair loss but can be treated with a lotion from your GP.

• Alopecia areata is a baldness which can affect all the hair on the body, including the eyebrows, with the cause often never found but thankfully the hair may regrow.

• Chronic illness can affect hair growth and a sustained fever may cause marked hair loss.

• Chemotherapy for cancer can sometimes cause hair loss but radiotherapy only rarely does so.

• Too frequent use of permanent-waving chemicals, or of shampoos or lotions, especially those containing alcohol, may cause dryness, but the jury is still out over actual hair loss.

• Thyroid gland under activity (myxoedema).

• There is no evidence that you can lose all the hair on your head from a fright.

3 There are drugs which block the conversion of testosterone to its dihydroxy form involved in male pattern baldness. Women can also be treated with these drugs but with less success. Unfortunately they are not available on the NHS and their lifetime cost may make you tear your hair out.

4 It may be sexy on Bruce Willis, but hair loss in a women can be devastating. As with men, short hair can look better – if it happens to your partner, treat her to a visit to a really good hairdresser.

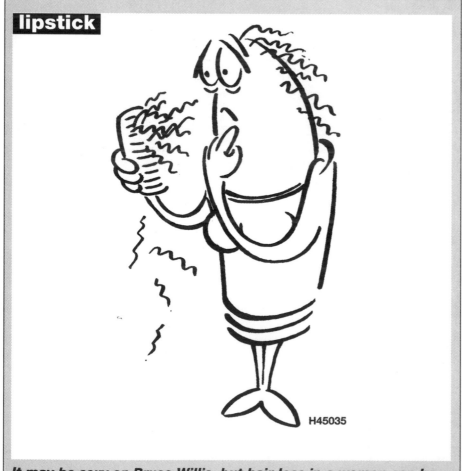

lipstick

H45035

It may be sexy on Bruce Willis, but hair loss in a women can be devastating

8 Hormone replacement therapy

1 Times change. With a life expectancy of around 35 years most women during the industrial revolution never actually experienced the menopause. Now the average woman lives for about 30 years after the menopause during which women are liable to progressive loss of bone strength (osteoporosis) and an increasing risk of heart attacks and strokes. Studies have shown that post-menopausal women taking HRT may have significant physical and other advantages over those not taking HRT.

2 Less certain than its role in preventing osteoporosis is the claim for preventing coronary heart disease. HRT is often mentioned in connection with the common menopausal symptoms such as hot flushes, night sweats, mood swings and depression. These are very unpleasant but they are not likely to continue for very long and there is no very clear medical evidence that these symptoms are necessarily due to oestrogen deficiency. Oestrogens are, however, widely prescribed for them and many people are convinced that they help.

3 The three really important problems affecting a high proportion of post-menopausal women are loss of bone strength; the rising risk of the arterial disease atherosclerosis; and vaginal dryness and shrinkage with a resulting increase in urinary infections. Loss of sex drive may also be a problem.

4 You never hear of men having a womenopause, do you?

5 Definite advantages of HRT:

• After the menopause, 3 to 5 per cent of the mass of bone is lost every year because of the lack of oestrogen. The normal rate after age 40 is 0.3 to 0.5 per cent per year. Ten or 20 years after menopause, a woman's bones may be brittle and can break easily after a fall, with serious results. This is one of the main reasons for hip replacement and hip repair.

• As result, the incidence of bone fractures on minor trauma rises steeply with increasing age. Spinal column fractures, spinal curvature from bone softening, hip fractures and forearm

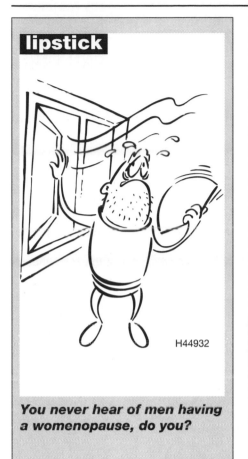

lipstick

You never hear of men having a womenopause, do you?

fractures become extremely common. Osteoporosis causes fractures on minimal exposure to damage in at least a quarter of elderly women. These fractures often have serious consequences.

• Women generally have a much lower risk of heart disease and stroke before menopause than men do. After the menopause, this risk soon rises to almost equal the risk in men. Most women think that breast cancer is their biggest killer in older age, not so. Women die more commonly from heart disease. Earlier trials suggested that women on HRT have about half the risk of coronary heart disease of those not on it. There is also the undeniable fact that HRT reduces the levels of the dangerous blood cholesterol carriers (low-density lipoproteins) by 10 to 14 per cent, and raised the levels of safe cholesterol carriers (high-density lipoprotein) by 7 to 8 per cent. These changes are known to be associated with a reduced risk of atherosclerosis and heart attacks.

• What we know is that HRT does not affect the progression of established

atherosclerosis or coronary heart disease, nor does it reduce the death rate in women who already have coronary heart disease. There is also some evidence that HRT does not, in fact, reduce heart attacks and strokes in women with no pre-existing disease.

Sandy bits

6 On the big plus side, there are few doubts about the value of local oestrogens in preventing and even treating post-menopausal vaginal dryness and atrophy (shrinkage). It is, of course, a major cause of post-menopausal sexual difficulty and will often make sexual intercourse virtually impossible, with visions of sandpaper meeting sandpaper.

7 The vaginal skin depends on oestrogen for the health, thickness and lubrication of its surface layer. Oestrogen lack causes it to thin and become dry. After the menopause there is also a change in the kind of bacteria normally found in the vagina and a change in the vaginal acidity. Live natural yoghurt (applied not eaten) helps restore this balance while lubricants can reduce the need for walking like John Wayne.

8 Post-menopausal vaginal atrophy is also linked to urinary tract symptoms such as having to go to the toilet more often (frequency, urgency and incontinence) which may often be due to oestrogen deficiency rather than urinary infection. Many doctors routinely prescribe oestrogen-containing vaginal creams, pessaries or rings to treat post-menopausal vaginal atrophy.

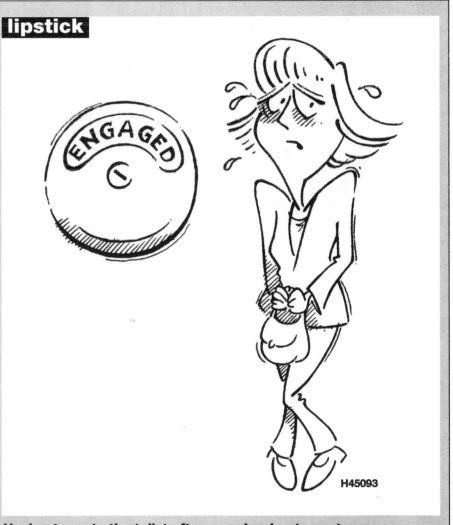

lipstick

Having to go to the toilet often may be due to oestrogen deficiency rather than urinary infection

2

Now the bad news

9 Women on HRT with oestrogen alone have a small but definite increase in the risk of cancer of the lining of the womb (endometrial cancer). The increase is 8 to 10 times in women who use oestrogen-only HRT for 10 years or more. The effect of this is that for every 10,000 women, there will be an additional 46 cases of endometrial cancer each year.

10 HRT increases the risk of deep vein thrombosis and embolism by a factor of 2 to 3.5. This applies whether oestrogen alone or the combined therapy is taken. The effect of this increase is that for every 10,000 women on HRT there will be 2 additional cases per year over the incidence in the same number of women not on HRT.

11 Current evidence also suggests that there is a significantly increased risk of breast cancer and this is being taken increasingly seriously by doctors.

Decision

12 At the end of the day only the woman herself can make the final decision based on good advice. It is fair to say that all the evidence is that it can, with relative safety, be taken for a few years, and longer in women who start a menopause unusually early.

13 However, HRT really should not be taken by a woman who:

• Has unusual vaginal bleeding that hasn't been investigated.

• Has had breast or womb cancer, as dormant traces of the disease could theoretically be stimulated by HRT.

• Has had a stroke or deep-vein thrombosis, or has high blood pressure.

• Has severe liver or gallbladder disease.

14 Perhaps most importantly HRT must not be used if there is any chance of being pregnant (still the most common reason for periods to stop, and a possibility for up to two years after the start of the menopause).

Treatment options

15 Because of the danger from womb cancer, oestrogen is taken alone (without progesterone), and continuously, only by women whose womb has been removed by hysterectomy.

16 Progesterone is given with oestrogen to women with a womb, as oestrogen alone could raise the risk of cancer of the lining of the womb (endometrial carcinoma). It can be given for 14 days a month (cyclical therapy), which results in a light period each month after it is stopped.

17 Combined preparations are now available that give a period only every three months. Truly continuous preparations are recommended only for women who have not had a period for a year; they produce no periods.

18 HRT can be given as daily tablets; in skin patches; as a rub-in gel; and as a pellet implanted under the skin every six months. Local oestrogen therapy for vaginal action only can be given as a vaginal pessary, cream, or ring. HRT does not suit everyone and if several different types of HRT have been tried with side-effects causing more problems than the menopause did, then it is better to stop. Some women are also allergic to the skin patches rather than the hormone they contain.

9   Itchy anus (pruritus)

1 There can be few things more satisfying than giving the bum a good scratching, and an itchy bottom is more common in adults than we like to admit or do anything about in public. Thankfully, there are very few serious conditions which cause the itch although it can be embarrassing.

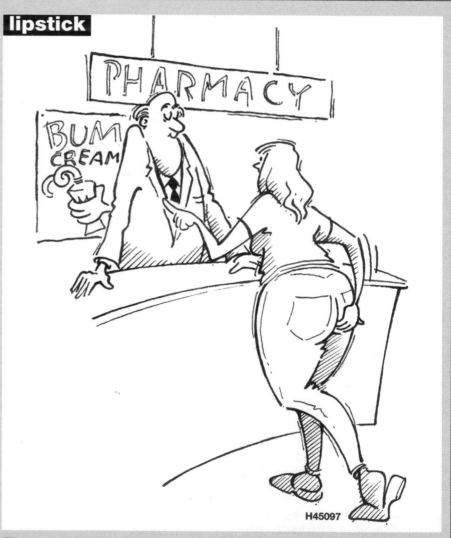

lipstick

There can be few things more satisfying than giving the bum a good scratching

Symptoms

2 A great deal depends on what is causing the itch.

3 Threadworms lay their eggs in a ring around the anus at night which irritates the skin. This is deliberate as the infected person then scratches the itch and later inevitably either passes the eggs on to someone else or passes them back into their own mouth to make things even worse. The fine white worms can be seen in the motions.

4 Piles, tears around the anus from straining with constipation and irritation from excessive wiping after diarrhoea will make the anus itchy shortly after passing a motion.

5 Coarse toilet paper or failing to clean properly are common causes.

6 In most case the cause is unknown and is probably due to dampness and heat. This is more noticeable at night when there are less distractions.

Causes

7 Most causes will not be found and will be simple, such as warm weather.

Prevention

• Wear loose cotton underwear.
• Eat a high fibre diet to prevent constipation causing small tears around the anus or piles.
• Use damp toilet paper first then dry paper after passing a motion.
• Avoid harsh toilet paper and strong soaps.
• Loose cotton underwear isn't exactly sexy but you can go back to the thongs after treatment. It's a good idea to use wet wipes whenever you go to the loo.

Complications

8 Constant itching can cause infection which only makes the itching worse. If it is caused by threadworms they almost always will be passed to other members of the family.

Self care

9 Creams are available from the pharmacist to ease the itching and there are sprays which the doctor can prescribe.

10 Check the motions for worms, particularly if there is a night time itch. Worming medicines act swiftly and effectively but all the family should take it.

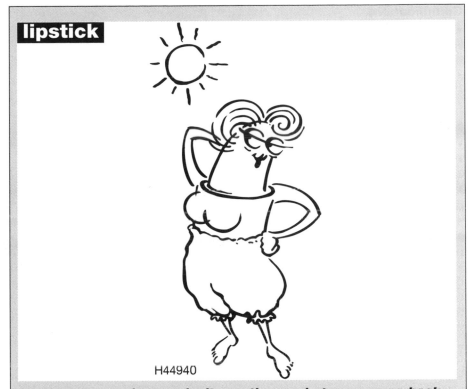

lipstick

H44940

Loose cotton underwear isn't exactly sexy but you can go back to the thongs after treatment

10 Lice & crabs

1 Reading this will have you scratching just the way people yawning make you follow suit. These tiny parasites live on any hairy bits of the body. Head lice live in scalp hair, body lice will live in the armpits while crab lice prefer the groin but will survive quite happily in the eyebrows. Contrary to the myth, they do not survive by sucking blood from the skin. Instead they chomp on dead skin. The itchiness comes from scratching with fingernails. Female lice lay eggs every day. The eggs hatch in eight to 10 days. Social status means nothing to lice. They are very common amongst children and infestation has nothing to do with dirty living. They are completely harmless, if terribly irritating.

Symptoms

• Itchiness is a common first symptom.
• The adults can be seen crawling about in the hair.
• Nits can be seen attached to the hair shafts.

• Inflamed areas around the hair shafts are common, usually caused by scratching.

Causes

2 There is only one source of lice and crabs; other people and their clothes. You can pick up similar parasites from pets but they don't survive long on people.

3 Teachers and doctors often pick up these fellow travellers, so do children.

4 It is possible to catch them from second hand clothes or wearing other people's clothes but much less common than direct contact with other people. Dry cleaning and washing generally gets rid of the adults and their eggs (nits).

Prevention

• Avoid sharing hats, scarves or combs.
• Act promptly when warned of infection in the child's school.
• Check all the family, lice like to move around and meet people.
• Lice are easily caught from others, so avoid spreading lice by treating the whole family.

Complications

• Although they are bad neighbours, lice and crabs do not cause any serious harm.

• Scratching may cause secondary infection which may need antibiotic cream.

Self care

• Keep the hair clean.

• Comb the hair while wet regularly with a fine-toothed comb.

• Use a conditioner. This helps to prevent the spread of lice.

• Ask a pharmacist for the most suitable lotion. There will be a local policy on the treatment of head lice.

• The most effective treatment is daily combing with a nit comb followed by chemical lotions. Organophosphates are the mainstay of lice treatments but there is concern that they be dangerous if used too often in young children. If in doubt, use only conditioner and nit comb.

• As lice can stay alive for two days when they are not on a person, thoroughly clean clothes and hats which have been worn, as well as combs and brushes.

11 Liver disease

1 Although men suffer more from liver disease, it is also on the increase in women. Alcohol abuse is by far the greatest cause along with a worrying increase in viral hepatitis. Cirrhosis is the deterioration of the liver due to gradual internal scarring of its tissues. This destroys the ability of the liver to carry out its numerous and vital functions such as detoxifying the blood. Many drugs and toxins such as alcohol are broken down in the liver. It also produces hormones and albumin to control body functions and maintain the correct balance of water in the blood and cells of the body. Very importantly it produces many of the clotting factors which stop bleeding. Damage to the liver, therefore, can have a very wide range of effects and symptoms.

Symptoms

2 Such is the level of reserves of this, the largest internal organ of the body, it can be suffering damage without any signs. At most in the early stages there are only mild symptoms. As the damage builds up there can be vomiting, weight loss, general malaise, indigestion and swelling of the abdomen. As the clotting factors are disrupted, bruising becomes easier to produce, with frequent nosebleeds and blood in the urine. Small red spider like spots can appear on the upper chest arms and face. If the liver is not allowed to recover or the damage continues it cannot break down the haemoglobin from worn out red blood cells and this pigment builds up in the skin and white of the eyes. This jaundice can be mistaken in the early stages for a

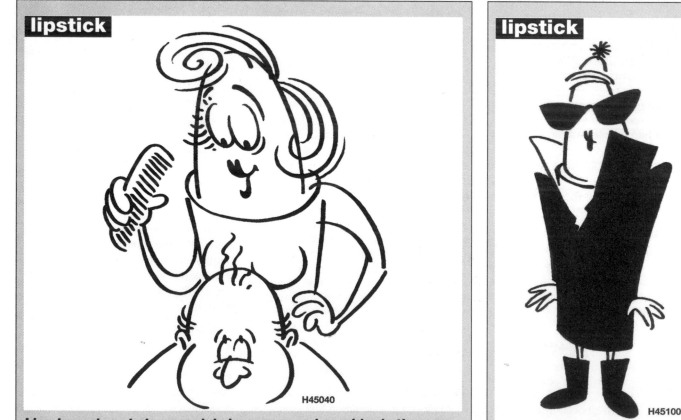

Lice love clean hair – special shampoos and combing's the way to beat them. Come on darlin', let me comb your hair – you know you like it!

I did think a suntan in January was a bit odd...

suntan but as it progresses the sallow colour deepens and is seen in the white of the eyes.

Causes

3 There are many causes which include chronic alcohol abuse, malnutrition, and infections such as a virus causing hepatitis.

Prevention

4 Moderation in alcohol consumption is the single greatest protection from liver disease. Vaccination against hepatitis in all forms makes sense especially if there

is a high risk. Travel to countries with such risks often requires prior vaccination.

Complications

5 The good news is that the liver has a remarkable ability to regenerate even when a large proportion of the organ has been damaged. This can take a long time and obviously depends on the avoidance of whatever was causing the damage in the first place. Unfortunately total liver failure is fatal, but liver transplantation is increasingly a possibility.

Self care

6 Protein is also broken down in the liver, so if it is damaged toxic residues from incomplete protein metabolism build up and further inhibit the remaining normal function of the liver. Big juicy steaks are out. Taking supplements such as vitamin B complexes may help protect the liver but this is controversial.

12 Malignant melanoma

See Chapter 7.

13 Maternal Rubella

1 Although German Measles (Rubella) is relatively mild and harmless viral infection in children or adults it can have devastating effects on the early pregnancy. The more serous effects on the developing baby include:
• Heart defects.
• Cataracts.
• Deafness.
• Neurological defects.
• Mental retardation.
• Bone and joint defects.
2 Although the severity of effect varies greatly, with many children suffering no apparent harm, around a quarter of babies infected while in the womb will show some problems by the age of two years. Women who are not immune should be particularly careful to avoid contact with any possible case and should be immunized as soon as the pregnancy is over.
3 Such is the danger of malformation, any non-immune pregnant women developing a rash and swollen glands in the back of the neck early in pregnancy should get themselves checked to discover whether the condition is Rubella. Termination is an option and needs discussion with professionals who can give you the facts objectively. Obviously all girls and boys should be immunised to prevent this happening in the first place.

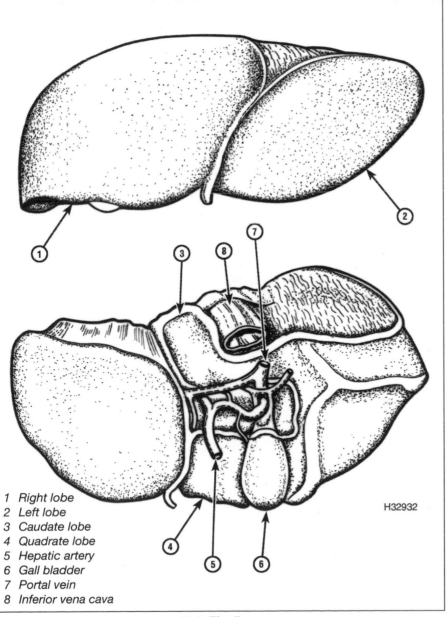

1 Right lobe
2 Left lobe
3 Caudate lobe
4 Quadrate lobe
5 Hepatic artery
6 Gall bladder
7 Portal vein
8 Inferior vena cava

H32932

11.1 The liver

14 Mouth ulcers

1   The mouth is one of the most nerve-rich parts of the body which is why a small ulcer can feel like a volcano. Sadly, they are very common although the vast majority are harmless and will clear on their own. Unfortunately some ulcers may be more serious and need a doctor's attention. There are different types of ulcer the commonest of which is the aphthous ulcer seen more often in teenagers or women just before their period. Teeth with jagged edges or badly fitting dentures will also cause ulcers, particularly on the gums and cheeks.

Symptoms

2   Aphthous ulcers are small, white and usually less than pin-head sized with a red border and despite being particularly painful will disappear within a week or so. They usually appear on the inside of the lower lip or inside the cheeks.

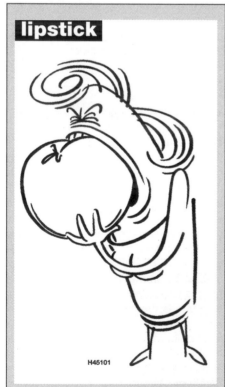
lipstick

H45101

If an apple a day doesn't work then maybe we all need a regular visit to the dentist. Don't be a baby – you know it makes sense!

Drinking something hot or acidic like orange juice usually makes their presence felt. Ulcers from teeth or dentures are usually larger and get bigger rather than disappear. Any ulcer which fails to get better should be seen by a dentist or doctor.

Causes

3   Aphthous ulcers appear spontaneously but more often during stress or being run down. Constant rubbing from a tooth, filling, dental plate or dentures will also cause an ulcer. Tongue and mouth cancer is extremely rare in young people.

Prevention

4   Except for correct maintenance and checking of dentures there is no real prevention from mouth ulcers. Some doctors feel that vitamin C helps reduce mouth ulcers but the evidence is thin on the ground. Regular dental check ups will ensure any persistent ulcer is sorted out.

Complications

5   Ulcers from teeth or dentures can become infected making eating even more painful.

Self care

6   Aphthous ulcers may respond to salt water rinses but it should not be swallowed and the salt rinse washed out with fresh water afterwards. A mild cortisone cream will speed the recovery. Avoid antibacterial mouthwashes or lozenges which at best are useless and may even make matters worse. Make sure dentures fit properly. Avoid using gels which numb the pain as it will only disguise the extent of the problem. Any ulcer which has not gone within 2-3 weeks, needs a doctor or dentist's attention.

15 Obesity

1   Obesity is the term used when a person's excess weight is enough to cause significantly increased risk of ill health. Obesity leads to a variety of illnesses and conditions, and on average will cause a 5-year reduction in a woman's life, commonly because of diabetes, heart disease and stroke. An obese woman is around four times as likely to have a heart attack, and can be 30 times more likely to get diabetes, than a woman of normal weight. It also causes arthritis, increases the risk of fatal accidents, asthma, chronic bronchitis, liver disease, kidney disease and depression. Although some overweight women are lucky, and live to a ripe old age without any major problem, most obese women will discover that chronic ill health is in store for them, and the risk is greater the fatter they become. Being fat isn't just a cosmetic problem; it isn't just how you look, its how you feel, how much energy and life you've got, and how much life you may lose because of illness.

Weight and Cancer

2   Being overweight or obese also causes cancer. Nobody would disagree that smoking leads to cancer; but the connection with obesity is less obvious, despite the fact that obesity causes more different types of cancer than smoking, so in some ways is more dangerous. 1 in 10 cancers are obesity related, and around 1 in 7 of all cancer deaths in the over 50s are caused by obesity, according to a study of nearly 1 million Americans in 2003. Smoking cigarettes causes a large number cancer deaths, but obesity isn't far behind, and we're set to see an epidemic of weight-related cancers in the next 20 years because of the current epidemic of obesity. The evidence is clear that just as stopping smoking is important if you want to live to see your grandchildren growing up, so is losing weight. The extremely good news is that by losing weight, the extra chances of getting cancer reduce and disappear.

Size Does Matter!

3   There are many different places a person can store fat; arms, legs, backside; but the place that matters most is the belly. Someone once compared fat people to either apples or pears. 'Pears' are typically women with big rears and thighs, and 'apples' are often men with big bellies.

Seeing Your Doctor

4   Obesity causes 30,000 deaths in the UK every year, and 18 million working days are lost because of fat-related illness. In America over one third of the population is obese, and 300,000 people

Height / weight chart – Imperial (height in inches, weight in pounds)

Height	Underweight	Healthy weight	Overweight	Obese
63	up to 113	113 – 141	141 – 169	169 plus
64	up to115	115 – 144	144 – 173	173 plus
65	up to 121	121 – 151	151 – 182	182 plus
66	up to 124	124 – 155	155 – 186	186 plus
67	up to127	127 – 159	159 – 191	191 plus
68	up to 132	132 – 165	165 – 197	197 plus
69	up to 135	135 – 168	168 – 202	202 plus
70	up to 140	140 – 174	174 – 209	209 plus
71	up to143	143 – 178	178 – 214	214 plus
72	up to 147	147 – 184	184 – 221	221 plus
74	up to 155	155 – 194	194 – 233	233 plus
75	up to 159	159 – 199	199 – 238	238 plus

Height / weight chart – metric (height in metres, weight in kilograms)

Height	Underweight	Healthy weight	Overweight	Obese
1.60	up to 51	51 – 64	64 – 77	77 plus
1.63	up to 52	52 – 65	65 – 79	79 plus
1.65	up to 55	55 – 69	69 – 83	83 plus
1.68	up to 56	56 – 70	70 – 84	84 plus
1.70	up to 58	58 – 72	72 – 87	87 plus
1.73	up to 60	60 – 75	75 – 89	89 plus
1.75	up to 61	61 – 76	76 – 92	92 plus
1.78	up to 64	64 – 79	79 – 95	95 plus
1.80	up to 65	65 – 81	81 – 97	97 plus
1.83	up to 67	67 – 84	84 – 100	100 plus
1.88	up to 70	70 – 88	88 – 106	106 plus
1.91	up to 72	72 – 90	90 – 108	108 plus

die each year because of it, and we're following in their footsteps. Its not just 'being fat' that kills you, it's the illness you get because you're fat that causes the trouble. This is likely to be diabetes or heart disease, but if you're unlucky it will be cancer.

5 BMI (Body Mass Index), an indicator of body fat, is important because the higher the BMI gets, the more fat proportion in the body and thus the higher risk of illness. A BMI of 30 or above is technically obese. This is a horrible word, but is used with great care, because it means that there is fat enough to cause illness, and possibly an early grave. BMI is calculated as follows:

a) *Using pounds and inches. Multiply your weight in pounds by 700 and divide that figure by the square of your height in inches. For example, if you're 68 inches tall and weigh 185 pounds, your BMI is*
185 x 700 ÷ (68 x 68 = 4624) = 28.

b) *Using kilograms and metres. Divide your weight in kilograms by the square of your height in metres. This means if you're 1.78 metres tall and weigh 78 kg, your BMI is*
78 ÷ (1.78 x 1.78 = 3.2) = 24.4.

2

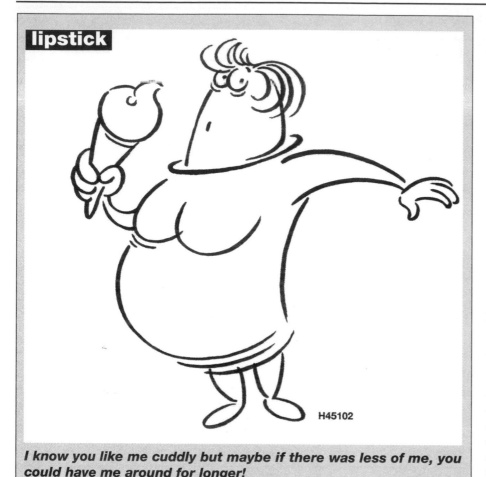

lipstick

H45102

I know you like me cuddly but maybe if there was less of me, you could have me around for longer!

How Does Obesity Cause Cancer?

6 Obesity causes a number of different illnesses, including cancer, in a number of different ways, which are extremely complicated, and not yet fully understood by scientists. What we do know is that fat people don't deal with sugar very well. Just as a car engine uses petrol, muscles use sugar for fuel; our fuel tank is the blood stream where sugar circulates before being used; and when we run out of sugar we don't function well, so we fill the tank up by eating. Sugar doesn't just come from sweet stuff, our bodies also extract sugar from carbohydrates such as bread and pasta, to prevent the needle going onto 'empty'. Our muscles use a hormone called insulin, made in the pancreas, to extract the sugar from the blood, and the more sugar we have, the more insulin we need. Fat people have too much sugar in the blood and an increased resistance to the effects of insulin, so they need to overproduce insulin to deliver enough sugar to the muscles. So they end up having too much sugar AND too much insulin. The excess sugar can lead to diabetes, and the extra insulin has serious damaging effects of its own.

Toxic Waist

7 Insulin is a dangerous substance if you have too much of it; when it circulates in the blood, all the tissues of the body come into contact with it, and its toxic effects. So by being fat, a woman poisons herself; in obesity, the poison is made within the body, every minute of every day. Each tissue or organ of the body reacts in a different way to insulin: the kidneys retain too much salt in the blood, putting blood pressure up; our glands produce abnormal hormones, affecting sex drive and fertility; other organs such as the bowel react by becoming inflamed, and eventually developing cancer.

8 And there's more bad news. Fatty tissue doesn't just sit buried inside our abdomens doing nothing. Instead it acts like a lump of toxic waste buried in concrete in our countryside; it leaks hazardous chemicals into the water supply and wreaks havoc. These hazardous chemicals, one in particular called IGF-1, mixed together with insulin, are called 'Fat Toxins'.

Cancer of the Bowel

9 Cancer of the bowel is the third most common cancer in America, and one of the cancers most closely linked with obesity. Weight related bowel cancers usually occur in the large bowel or colon, at the far end of the gut, where the last part of the digestive process occurs, but can occur elsewhere in the bowel. Although related to obesity, cancer of the colon may cause unexplained weight loss, as well as a change in bowel habit, or sometimes the passage of blood or mucus with a motion.

10 Obesity causes colon cancer in two ways. One is the action of fat toxins on the cells of the bowel. The cells lining the gut are naturally lost and replaced very quickly, and such rapidly growing cells are susceptible to cancer-causing chemicals, like fat toxins. The other reason seems to be that some cancer-causing chemicals within our food are absorbed by fatty tissue, and trapped for a long time; because obese women store more fat, they store more of these carcinogens, leading to bowel cancer.

Breast and womb cancer

12 In women, hormone problems resulting from obesity can cause abnormalities of the ovaries, and a big increase in the risk of breast cancer, and cancer of the womb.

Cancer of the liver

13 When a person is obese she has too much fat inside the abdomen, which surrounds and wraps the internal organs, including the gut, even extending up to the heart. But the fat also turns up inside the liver. More often than not the liver manages to carry on doing its job despite the extra fat, but sometimes the fat causes the liver to malfunction in the same way as drinking too much alcohol does. In severe cases, as with alcohol, this leads to cirrhosis, liver failure, jaundice and sometimes liver cancer.

The risks are much greater if a person is both obese and a heavy drinker. Abnormalities in the liver can be picked up on blood tests, or on ultrasound examination. Obesity is also linked with gallstones and gallbladder cancer.

Cancer of the kidney

14 Cancer of the kidney, or renal cell carcinoma, is caused by the circulating fat toxins in obese people. The kidneys are extremely sensitive to these toxins, and also respond by retaining salt in the body, instead of removing it in the urine. This causes high blood pressure in the same way as eating too much salty food in our diet causes high blood pressure, so obese people in particular should limit the amount of salt they eat.

Cancer of the Oesophagus and Stomach

15 Cancer of the oesophagus causes difficulty in swallowing food, and can eventually block the food pipe altogether. Various different things make oesophageal cancer more likely, including drinking spirits, smoking, and heavily spiced food, but obesity has a role to play as well.

16 The lining of the oesophagus is sensitive, and protected from the strong acid produced by the stomach to digest food by a valve which opens and shuts to let food through. The oesophagus should only come into contact with the food we eat, and saliva. In obesity, the bulk of the fat around the abdomen actually squashes the stomach, forcing the contents up through the closed valve and into the foodpipe. This will initially cause symptoms of indigestion and heartburn, but if persistent and prolonged can lead to cancer. The top of the stomach, or cardia is also at risk of cancer because of the abnormal flow of acid. An obese person who also smokes or drinks spirits has a much greater risk.

Other cancers

17 The more that scientists come to understand the disease, the more fat toxins in the blood are being blamed for different cancers. The list of cancers linked to obesity now also include the pancreas, small bowel, throat, lymphoma, Hodgkin's disease, and gallbladder cancer.

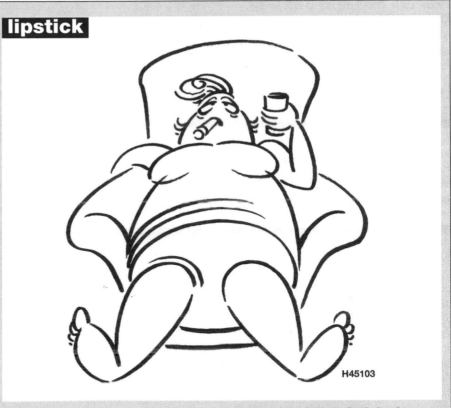

I drink and smoke because I'm depressed at being fat! And now I'm depressed about the health risks!! Oh alright then – let's work at losing weight and maybe we can deal with the lot.

Other risks

18 As well as actually being responsible for some cancers, obesity acts as an obstacle in the fight against cancer at every step of the way, whether or not a particular tumour is caused by obesity:

• It makes it more difficult for a person to discover the early signs of cancer; it's harder to find a lump if its hidden by surplus flesh.

• The symptoms of cancer may be masked by symptoms of obesity; breathlessness due to a lung tumour may be mistaken for unfitness because of being overweight, or bone pain may be put down to aching joints or arthritis, when it may be because of a bony tumour.

• It is more difficult for the doctor to perform a thorough examination and pick up subtle signs of cancer if hampered by a pillow of fat. The doctor may want to check for enlargement of the liver, or a lump in the bowel, which if missed could allow the disease to get worse and spread.

• X-rays, ultrasounds or other tests may be less accurate in an obese person, because the image may be blurred in the presence of too much fat.

• Any operation needed to help diagnose, or even to remove a malignant growth will be far more complex and less likely to succeed in an obese patient. The operation will take longer, be technically more challenging, and there will be more blood lost. The anaesthetist will have to use more gas, and will have to be careful to prevent complications of breathing including pulmonary embolism and infection. The recovery after surgery is more hazardous, and there is risk of pressure sores, deep vein thrombosis and wound infection. It is harder for nurses and families to care for an obese person without risking injury especially back injuries through lifting.

• It can be difficult to work out and apply the correct doses of anti-cancer drugs in obese people because fatty tissue absorbs some drugs like a sponge, making them less effective.

2

How can the risk of cancer be reduced?

19 The risk of obesity-related cancer can only be significantly reduced by losing weight, but the good news is that by losing 10% of their weight, women can almost halve their risk of dying from these diseases.

20 As well as varying lifestyle in order to lose weight there are specific dietary and exercise recommendations relating to cancer risk. A wide variety of fruit and vegetables should be consumed to help protect against cancer, because a low intake seems to increase risk, especially of bowel and stomach cancer. Additional fibre should be included in the diet to lower the risk of colon and pancreatic cancer, but a large intake of red meat may exaggerate the risk, so some experts suggest it should be limited. Diet should be low in saturated fat.

21 High levels of physical activity are known to provide some protection against colon cancer. The International Agency for Research on Cancer suggest that 13-14% of cases of colon cancer are attributable to sedentary lifestyle, although some studies suggest a 70% reduction in cases of colon cancer in active individuals. For protection against cancer, any exercise will do, as long as enough energy is expended, so a short burst of vigorous exercise has as much benefit as prolonged moderate exercise. For the purposes of weight loss, however, exercise should be brisk rather than vigorous, and in any case should be maintained as a permanent way of life. Women who are physically active have a substantial reduction in risk of breast cancer, so exercise as a family benefits everyone.

How to lose weight

22 Obesity is caused by taking in more energy as food than is burned off by activity. Some people seem to eat less than others and still gain weight, others can eat non-stop, and not gain an ounce, but that is just a fact of life. Another fact of life is that if you're obese you probably need to eat less and do more.

You Are What You Eat

23 Sometimes the answer is just to cut down on food; by reducing portion sizes, and trying to avoid snacks between meals; but sometimes the type of food has to change. It is important to have a well-balanced diet, containing protein, carbohydrate, and a certain amount of fat, but not too much. As a general rule, the sort of food that is high in fat, and bad for us, is the sort of food that looks bad for us, i.e., it's fairly obvious. Chips, crisps, fry-ups, pies, fatty meat, junk food, many take-aways and chocolate are good examples. Foods like this should only be eaten as occasional treats, and not eaten regularly as they contain saturated fats, and are very high in calories, which cause weight gain. There's plenty of enjoyable food that is healthy and can be eaten without guilt. Curries and stir-fries can be extremely healthy without spoiling their appeal; meat and fish, fruit, bread and pasta, can be eaten freely, as long as they're prepared healthily (which is just as easy as preparing them unhealthily).

'You Should Get Out More!'

24 Physical activity is essential in the fight against obesity and against cancer in particular. It also protects against high blood pressure, high cholesterol and heart disease, so a sitting-down job, watching too much TV, or driving short journeys instead of walking, needs a re-think. Physical activity can be increased as part of the daily routine, without going down to the local gym, although sport and swimming is beneficial. The ideal intensity of exercise to lose weight is brisk enough for breathlessness, and work up a sweat, but doesn't prevent talking; so brisk walking fits the bill. Small changes can make a big difference, for example walking up the stairs or escalators, instead of using the lift. Walking to work instead of using the bus, or walking that bit further to buy a (healthy) lunch. Gardening is a great way to take some exercise. Even housework counts. Any exercise helps, even something as simple as standing up when using the telephone.

25 To stay healthy, a person should do at least 30 minutes of exercise every day, in one spell or in combination, but a woman needing to lose weight, or maintain the weight they've lost, must do as much as possible, even 60-90 minutes per day. Doing unaccustomed exercise should be done carefully without overdoing it.

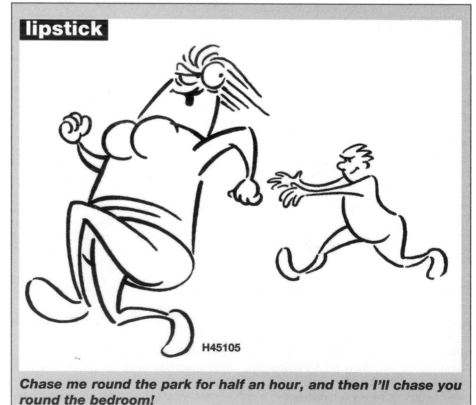

lipstick

H45105

Chase me round the park for half an hour, and then I'll chase you round the bedroom!

How to get help

26 There are many ways of seeking help and most are directed toward women. Many slimming clubs like Rosemary Conley, Weight Watchers and Slimming World will accept men as well so it can be a joint effort. Local GP surgeries often have special clinics where the practice nurse or doctor will help. They may provide information and encouragement or refer to a dietician, but if necessary there are safe and effective weight loss medications prescribed by GPs. A new drug is soon to be launched which helps stop the craving for food. Help and counselling by a therapist is useful for some people, others may need referring to a hospital specialist, or even be advised to undergo an operation, which nowadays is done by keyhole surgery. Many pharmacists now provide weight loss advice.

16 Osteoarthritis

1 This degenerative joint disorder involves damage to the cartilaginous bearing surfaces and sometimes damage of the ends of the bones involved in the joint. It is related to age. Many people of 30 show early osteoarthritic changes, and by the age of 65 about 80 per cent of people have some X-ray or other evidence of the disorder. Osteoarthritis most commonly involves the spine, the knee joints and the hip joints.

Symptoms

2 Pain is at first intermittent and then becomes more frequent. Joint movement becomes progressively more limited, at first because of pain and muscle spasm, but later because the joint capsule becomes thickened and less flexible. Movement may cause creaking. As the condition gradually gets worse stiffness increases and there is progressive reduction in the range through which the affected joints can be moved without pain.

Causes

3 While the cause of osteoarthritis is unknown it is commonly associated with injury. Being overweight makes osteoarthritis significantly worse.

4 There may be a number of factors including:
- Injury.
- Excessive pressure from obesity.
- Overuse of certain joints.
- Infection.
- Damage to the joint nerve supply.
- Other joint diseases such as gout or rheumatoid arthritis.

5 There is also evidence of a genetic factor in osteoarthritis.

Diagnosis

6 The diagnosis depends on things such as:
- Any family history of any similar joint disorder.
- When the symptoms started.
- The location of the pain.
- The severity of pain.
- Any time of day or activity when pain is worse.

7 In severe cases an X ray examination can be useful.

Prevention

8 Avoiding weight gain and using exercises to maintain muscle strength around the knee help to reduce problems in osteoarthritis.

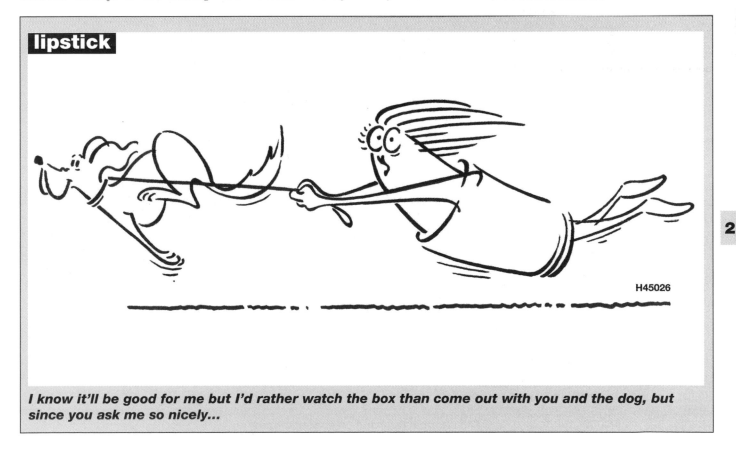

lipstick

H45026

I know it'll be good for me but I'd rather watch the box than come out with you and the dog, but since you ask me so nicely...

Treatment

9 Weight reduction can in itself, greatly reduce the severity of symptoms. An exercise program designed to improve the general health and the health of affected joints is also helpful.

10 Immobilization, on the other hand, is dangerous and can speed the progress and worsen the outlook of the disease.

11 In osteoarthritis, drug treatment is of relatively minor importance because inflammation is not an important part of the process and infection is not involved. That leaves pain control. Aspirin, or one of the other non-steroidal anti-inflammatory drugs (NSAIDs) is often all that is required to relieve pain. Newer drugs are available which have less effect on the stomach lining, one of the problems with aspirin and older anti-inflammatory drugs.

12 Joint replacement surgery is considered only as a last resource but is considered before total loss of function occurs. A large amount of surgical experience of hip and knee replacement for osteoarthritis has now been obtained, and the results are usually remarkably good. Other osteoarthritis joints can also be replaced.

17 Osteoporosis (thin bones)

1 Far from simply being like scaffolding or girders on to which all the soft living parts of the body are attached, bone is in fact constantly developing and changing its shape to meet demands set on it. It has a large number of jobs some of which we only poorly understand.

2 Bone:
• Produces blood cells.
• Actively fights infection.
• Provides support and protection for vital organs.

3 For various reasons bone can loose its density and become light and easily broken. The constant replacement with new bone is affected by lack of exercise, some drugs and certain illness. Weightlessness in space is an extreme case of lack of demand on bones but even prolonged bed rest can also cause osteoporosis. It usually effects people in their 60s and older and is unfortunately

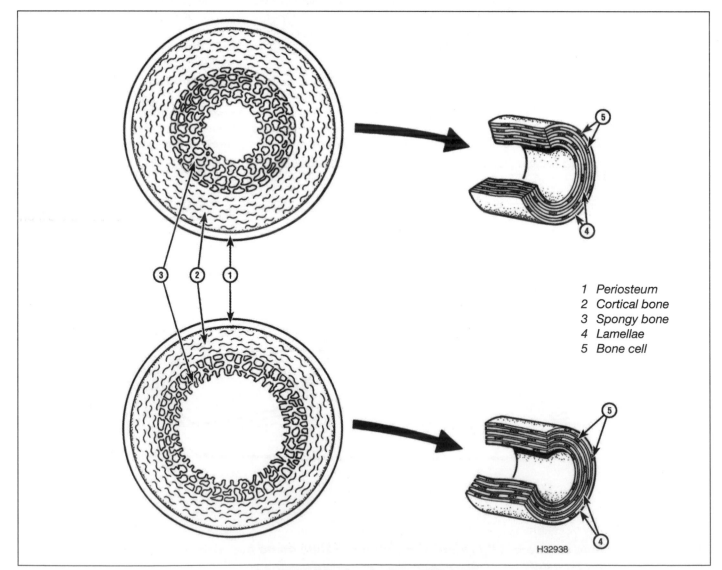

1 Periosteum
2 Cortical bone
3 Spongy bone
4 Lamellae
5 Bone cell

H32938

17.1 Normal (top) and osteoporitic bone

common in these age groups with over half affected to some degree. To a large extent keeping bone healthy and strong while younger pays great dividends later in life although the severity of osteoporosis is by no means the same for all women irrespective of their level of exercise in youth.

Symptoms

4 One of the major problems with detecting osteoporosis is the lack of any real warning signs. A chance X-ray for some other problem will often be the first time a person is aware of the potential problem. A sudden severe back pain may follow a collapsed vertebrae from osteoporosis. A simple fall can cause a broken hip. Often there is just a dull ache in the back or a loss of height noticed by women as a change in their clothing's fit.

Causes

5 There is no one single cause of osteoporosis but rather a complex battery of factors.

• Immobilisation (eg, bed rest or prolonged fixation in a cast).
• Lack of activity (a chronic illness or disability).
• Long term steroids (eg, for rheumatoid arthritis) will also tend to cause bone thinning. It is a matter of balancing the benefits of the treatment against the danger of osteoporosis.
• Hormone changes (eg, menopause or cancer of the pituitary gland).

Prevention

6 Hormone replacement therapy (HRT) is the mainstay of prevention but there is increasing concern over a possible link between it and breast cancer. Again, the benefits must be measured against this risk but HRT is now only being advised for short term treatment of menopause symptoms. There are drugs which when taken on a regular basis help prevent and possibly reverse osteoporosis.

Complications

7 Vertebrae collapse can cause pain in the back but also down into the legs and depending on the severity and location of the collapse, loss of sensation, muscle loss and difficulty controlling passing water. The most serious complication is the increased risk from fractures. Hip fractures are particularly common although with modern surgery this will not mean permanent disablement.

Self care

8 Regular activity, diet rich in calcium and vitamin D, and avoiding excessive strain on the back or leg bones are the best forms of prevention. Eating bread, milk, oily fish, fruit and vegetables makes supplements unnecessary but some people take extra calcium and vitamin D.

Further information

9 If you would like to know more, look at the contacts section at the back of this book, or contact:
National Osteoporosis Society
Tel: 01761 472721
Website: www.nos.org.uk

18 Psoriasis

1 Contrary to popular myth, psoriasis is not an infection and you cannot catch it from anyone else or their clothes. The silver flaky patches of skin are simply cells which are growing too fast. Around 2.5% (1 in 40) of the population suffer from psoriasis which does tend to run in families.

Symptoms

2 Psoriasis is classically found on the elbows and knees and the scalp but it thankfully tends to spare the face. In more severe cases it can also affect the soles of the feet, palms of the hands, small of the back and armpits. Characteristic psoriasis oval red patches are often covered with silver flaky scales which come away easily to expose the darker layers underneath. They are not usually itchy unless infected.

Causes

3 Psoriasis is an auto-immune condition where for some reason the body attacks itself. It is linked to other similar conditions such as rheumatoid arthritis. We now know there are various triggers which stimulate these areas of

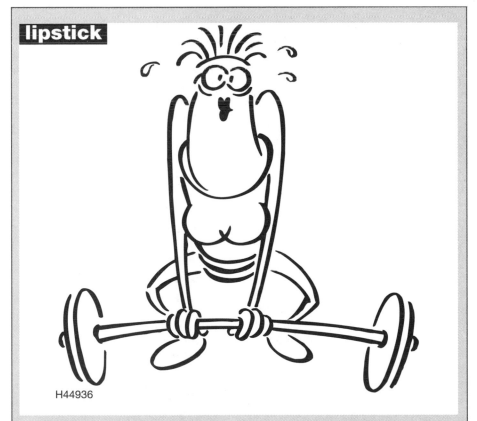

lipstick

H44936

Go to a gym together! Bone loading exercise really helps and has the added advantage of getting you slim and keeping you fit

2

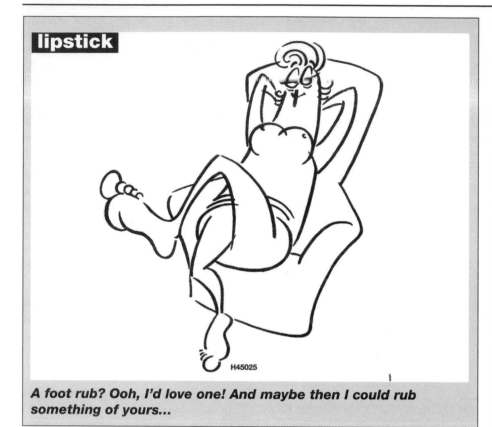

lipstick

A foot rub? Ooh, I'd love one! And maybe then I could rub something of yours...

skin to start growing too fast. Stress, overwork, changes in climate and even minor infections may enough to start the process off.

Prevention

4   It is difficult to suggest any effective form of protection from psoriasis outbreaks. Dealing effectively with stress through both relaxation and activity instead of resorting to alcohol may be valuable.

Complications

5   The rash is not dangerous unless it is very extensive or is infected. When the rash appears on the hands or feet it usually forms fluid filled blisters which resemble pus. There is no infection. A small proportion of psoriasis sufferers, 6-7% (less than one in 14), will experience joint pain resembling that of rheumatoid arthritis.

Self care

6   Care and treatment depends on the severity of the condition. Sunlight appears to help some people which is not surprising as ultra violet (UV) treatments have long been used with moderate success.

• Avoid strong soaps.
• Avoid overheating by wearing light cotton clothes.
• If the patches itch, use a moisturising cream but do not scratch them.
• Keep the skin moist with emollients.

7   Products from the pharmacist containing tar can be effective but do unfortunately stain clothes and need to be applied with care only to the affected skin.

19 Repetitive strain injuries – RSI (tendonitis)

1   Once we had tennis elbow, now with the explosion in computers repetitive strain injuries are more commonly associated with the wrists and fingers. In truth there were always a large number of people suffering from this often distressing and even debilitation condition. Musicians, particularly string instrumentalists, were well recognised to be at risk. Women are now suffering as much as men although the classic sufferers were carpenters and electricians. Nurses and secretaries can

suffer from tendon injury through repetitive movement.

Symptoms

2   RSI is hard to miss. Generally the pain gets steadily worse as the day goes on. During days off the pain eases only to come back again on return to work.

Causes

3   Tendons move inside a lubricated sheath not unlike a brake cable. Either from injury or repetitive movement the tendon becomes inflamed and moves as if it were 'rusty' and in need of oil. Worse still, this movement further inflames the sheath which tightens onto the tendon causing pain. In some severe cases small islands of bone form in the tendon itself which can completely obstruct any movement.

Prevention

4   Alternating repetitive movements with others helps reduce the risk. Use wrist exercises which are the 'opposite' of the normal repetitive movement. Every few minutes lifting the hands from the keyboard and flexing them downwards (they are normally held in a slightly backwards position, even at rest. Use a keyboard which keeps the hands in the correct position. Similarly for people using instruments or tools such as screwdrivers. Either spend a few minutes during a job rotating the wrists and elbow in the opposite direction to the repetitive movement. Consider an electric tool which eliminates the repetitive movement altogether.

Complications

5   Most people will find RSI simply a nuisance but for some it can mean the loss of employment and serious disability.

Self care

6   As well as the prevention exercises some people find great relief using anti-inflammatory drugs like ibuprofen. Gels that you rub in are of dubious value. Most of the relief comes from the massaging and warmth that it produces. Applying warm compresses along with gentle massage can ease the pain. Mixing paracetamol with an anti-inflammatory drug may give greater pain relief than when taken alone. Seriously consider a change of occupation if all else fails.

7 Steroid injection can give almost miraculous pain relief and restore normal function. Most doctors would be reluctant to repeat injections and it can be counter-productive in that the person returns to the work which caused the problem in the first place. Eventually the pain returns and there may be more serous damage.

20 Shingles

1 Few skin conditions can look as angry and irritating as shingles. It is caused by the same virus as that which causes chicken pox (varicella zoster virus, or VZV for short). It is particularly nasty if the immune system is not working properly, for instance during a severe illness, taking strong steroid medicines or while on treatment for cancer.

2 On the plus side, it is rare to develop shingles more than once.

Symptoms

• A tingling itchy feeling precedes a painful rash (this is important to recognise and act on quickly).

• It is only found on one side of the body (a sharp line is often seen with ones side completely free).

• Blisters then develop over the next few hours or days (these can be both painful and itchy).

• It usually follows a narrow strip of skin, common sites include the chest wall, face and upper legs (this follows the track of a nerve which supplies this part of the body).

• A general flu-like illness often accompanies the rash which may persist after the rash has gone.

Causes

3 The chicken pox virus sits dormant in the nerves, only to re-emerge at some time causing shingles. Obviously not having chicken pox in the first place is protective, but should you get it later in life it can be much worse, along with the possibility of shingles. It was once thought that you could not 'catch' shingles but this is now known not to be true, and for people who have problems with their immune system it can be very severe.

Prevention

4 Prevention is difficult, most people will develop the infection without realising where it came from. Chicken pox is highly contagious, especially amongst children.

Complications

5 Although sometimes very painful, shingles is rarely serious although people who are suffering from any condition or medicine which lowers their resistance to infection can be quite ill. Shingles during pregnancy should receive a doctor's attention.

6 One of the most serious (although thankfully rare) complications occurs if the infection spreads into the cornea of the eye. This can be predicted if the shingles spreads onto the tip of the nose as it may affect the eye and needs urgent medical attention.

7 Some people suffer from pain or sensitivity for a long time after the rash has gone. This is known as post-herpetic neuralgia. Ordinary pain killers may have little effect, in which case a doctor's advice should be sought.

Self care

• Antiviral medicines should be used immediately the tingling sensation is felt.

• Simple pain killers such as aspirin and paracetamol help but do not stop the shingles.

• Letting air reach the rash area helps stop it turning 'boggy' and developing a further bacterial infection.

• Scratching also increases the risk of further bacterial infection and can also cause scarring of the skin. Calamine lotion can ease the itchiness.

• Pain which follows the disappearance of the rash can be reduced by cooling the area with a bag of ice in a soft towel. Do not use frozen peas or ice directly on the skin and remove the pack after a few minutes.

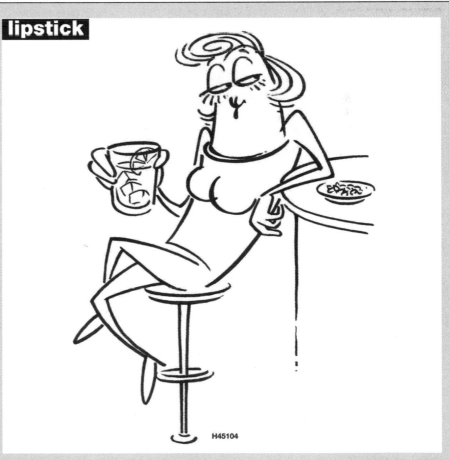

Ice in a towel and some ice in a G&T – now, that's what I call service!

2

21 Sinusitis

1 Women appear to suffer from sinusitis more than men. It is one of the few relatively harmless medical conditions which feels as though something very serious is happening. People are often convinced that they have a brain tumour or are having a stroke. Actually, although inflammation and infection of the hollow spaces of the face bones is extremely painful, it is rarely serious. Why some people suffer from repeated sinusitis while others avoid the problem altogether is a complete mystery.

Symptoms

2 People experience sinusitis in often very different ways and may depend on which of the sinuses – the hollow bone cavities – is affected. It is possible to have more than one sinus infected a the same time although this is much less common.
- The pain ranges from a persistent ache to full blown agony.
- It can feel like severe tooth ache or a headache with tenderness under the eyebrows.
- Generally the nose feels blocked up and there is nasal quality to the voice.

3 Although it can last for weeks, most will clear up within 7 days.

Causes

4 Some things are obvious. The sinuses may fail to drain though their ducts into the back of the nose and that it often follows a cold or allergic attack, but the exact cause is unknown.

Prevention

5 As the exact cause is unknown it is difficult to give good advice on prevention, but not smoking makes sense.

Complications

6 Serious complications such as infection spreading into the bone are now very rare not least thanks to antibiotics.

Self care

- Tackling the infection can take some time as there is only a poor penetration from the blood stream into the bony cavities. Pain relief while the treatment

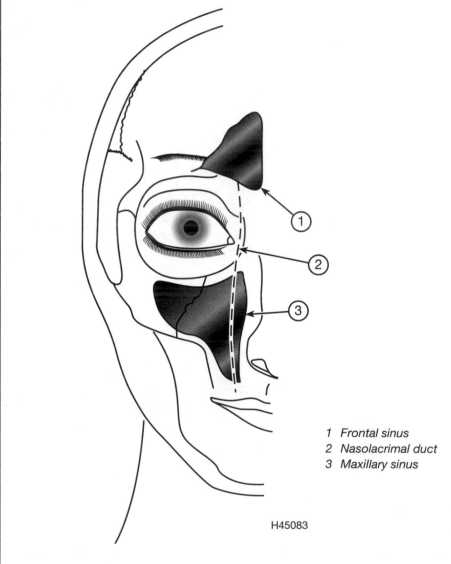

1 *Frontal sinus*
2 *Nasolacrimal duct*
3 *Maxillary sinus*

H45083

21.1 The face bones showing the position of the sinuses

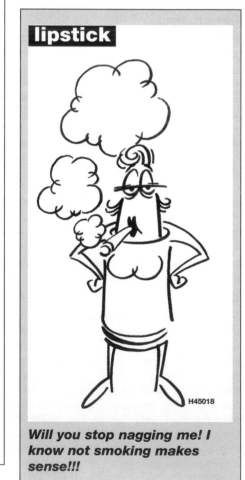

Will you stop nagging me! I know not smoking makes sense!!!

takes effect, therefore, is very important. Paracetamol or aspirin (not for children under 16 years) really can help.
• Decongestants may help initially but their overuse simply makes matters worse, particularly when they are stopped.
• Stop smoking.
• See your pharmacist for pain relief. If the pain persists phone your GP.
7 There are surgical treatments to flush out the sinuses but it is extremely unpleasant.

22 Skin cancer

See Chapter 7.

23 Sports injuries

1 Women are just as susceptible to sports injuries as are men. Obviously they play less contact sport so injuries such as fractures and head injuries are correspondingly less common. Whatever the sex, muscles, joints and bones are all very susceptible to damage when not treated properly. They all have limitations which when exceeded or prolonged overuse will cause damage, sometimes permanently.

Symptoms

2 While some injuries make their presence felt immediately, others show themselves as a gradual increase in pain on movement. This is typical of a repetitive strain injury or tendonitis ('Tennis elbow') but a snapped Achilles tendon can sound like a gun shot with immediate loss of power to the foot, severe pain and an inability to flex the ankle.
3 A ruptured meniscus (knee cartilage) invariably causes pain and swelling immediately or soon after it happens. It often happens when the foot is held on one position (say in a ski) while the leg is rotated. A 'locked' knee is a very obvious sign of internal damage such as a torn cartilage and must not be forced back into movement. This simply wrecks what is left of the normal knee structure.

4 Less serious but often just as painful is a sprain involving damage to tendons and ligaments stabilising or moving a joint. When these ligaments are either stretched or partly torn from the bone it causes pain and swelling with a restriction on movement. In all these cases the joint or muscle becomes hot and tender.

Causes

5 All sports injuries are caused either by a force exceeding that which the joint, muscle or tendon is designed to withstand, or prolonged repetitive movements. It is often the result of a twisting movement under great force (torn knee cartilages) or excessive force to an unprepared or inflexible tendon (torn Achilles tendon).

Prevention

6 No matter what sex or how fit, warming up before strenuous exercise is vital. Many women snap their Achilles through sudden activity especially if they are unused to exercise. Although some injuries are accidental and often unavoidable the damage is reduced by

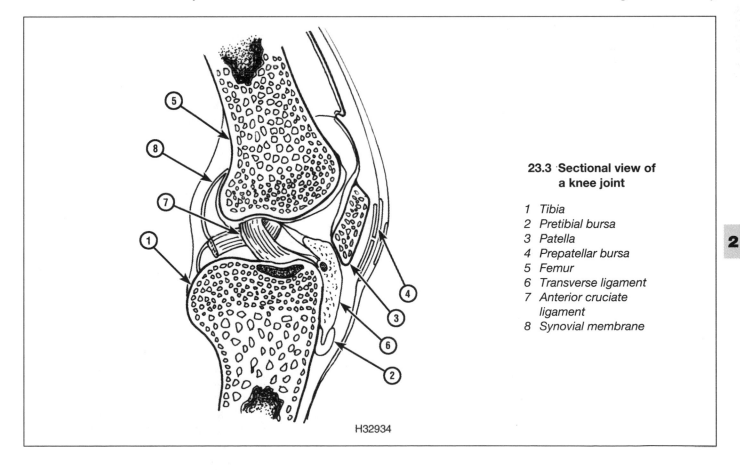

23.3 Sectional view of a knee joint

1 Tibia
2 Pretibial bursa
3 Patella
4 Prepatellar bursa
5 Femur
6 Transverse ligament
7 Anterior cruciate ligament
8 Synovial membrane

H32934

2

having the joint kept flexible through regular exercise. It will also heal much quicker because of the improved blood supply.

Complications

7 Many women with ankle injuries complain of osteoarthritis later in life. Although there is controversy over the link between osteoarthritis and sports injuries (such as hip problems in people who jog excessively on roads in poor footwear), common sense dictates that regular damage to a joint must impair its function eventually.

Self care

8 Many injuries do not require anything other than rest and time to sort them out. Physiotherapy may be required to restore normal function. Surgery is common for injuries such as torn knee cartilage or snapped tendons. Many of these treatments do not restore the normal state of the muscle, joint or tendon and there may be reduced movement or power.

8 Immediate first aid can help reduce pain and limit the permanent damage to the joint.

9 R.I.C.E is a system used by many first aiders and sports physiotherapists.

• R – Rest. Further movement will only make the damage worse. Once the initial inflammation has subsided gentle exercises help restore normal function.

• I – Ice. Cool the joint with bags of ice packed in cloth. This eases the pain and reduces the inflammation. Do not apply ice (or bags of frozen peas) directly to the skin. Remove the pack after 5 minutes maximum. Reapply every hour in the first 48 hours.

• C – Compression. An elastic bandage will help reduce swelling. Make sure it is well above and below the affected joint. Take it off at night.

• E – Elevation. Raise the limb and support it. This helps reduce swelling by draining the fluid away from the joint.

10 So called 'sports gels' containing anti-inflammatory drugs are of limited value as their penetration through the skin can be minimal, especially over large joints. But they do provide a benefit from the massage and warmth produced.

24 Sunburn

1 Although there is some controversy over the danger of exposure to too much sunlight, we do know that it can be harmful. Over the past few decades there has been a dramatic increase in the number of cases of malignant melanoma, a particularly nasty and potentially lethal skin cancer. Once considered rare, it is still increasing possibly due to the desire for sun-drenched holidays. Australia has been in the forefront of educating people over the dangers of sunbathing. You will be lucky to avoid being drenched in sun block from 'wardens' carrying back-pack sprayers on the watch for unprotected sunbathers on Australia's beaches.

Symptoms

2 The first sign of a burn is a reddening of the skin caused by blood vessels increasing in size to get rid of as much heat as possible (like a 'flush') Most people therefore, do not realise that they have badly burned themselves until later on in the day. At this stage damage is already being done to the skin. If the exposure to the sun continues the skin will form blisters just as with a scald. These blisters burst very quickly and the covering skin is then lost, exposing red skin beneath. If this is extensive, a large amount of body fluids can be lost.

Causes

3 Skin colour – the degree of pigmentation – is important as ultra violet light (UV) can penetrate the outer layers of skin, especially in fair skinned people. It heats and damages the lower layers causing skin loss. The only way the body can prevent further damage in the future is by increasing the amount of melanin, a black pigment, in the skin which

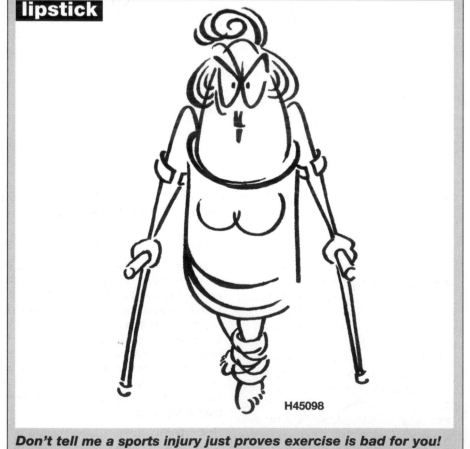

lipstick

H45098

Don't tell me a sports injury just proves exercise is bad for you! Help me get better and then chase me to the gym again – you know it makes sense!

prevents the sun from reaching the delicate lower skin layers. This is the 'suntan' we crave so much.

Prevention

4 There is now controversy over the effectiveness of sun block in preventing cancer but it probably makes sense to use a very strong sun block (factor 30 and over) effective against UVA and UVB. Better still, simply covering the body, especially the head, provides absolute protection. Even so some blouses and tops are so thin they are almost completely transparent to UV.

Complications

5 Like any burn, skin damaged by over-exposure to UV can scar. Long-term exposure to the sun causes the collagen network within the skin to become less flexible. This makes the skin lose its elasticity so it droops, folds and wrinkles very easily. Women are rapidly recognising the impact of sunburn on the aging process.

Self care

6 Treat sunburn like any other burn. There are lotions you can apply which will ease the pain but they cannot prevent the damage which is already done. Plenty of non-alcoholic fluids and staying out of the sun for a few days promotes skin repair and prevents further damage. Tepid baths ease the pain, warm baths make it worse and probably delay healing. Paracetamol will ease the pain and calamine lotion takes the sting out of the burn.

25 Sweat

1 With increased body temperatures there is an enhanced blood flow to the skin surface. When the temperature is low, blood vessels constrict to reduce blood flow and thus heat loss. Temperature is regulated by a special centre in the brain. Glands in the skin secrete moisture, which on evaporation cools the body surface. We tend to forget that the skin is really a waste disposal machine and gets rid of many toxins by this route. Dogs can taste the difference between 'clean' sweat and sweat contaminated by toxins such as

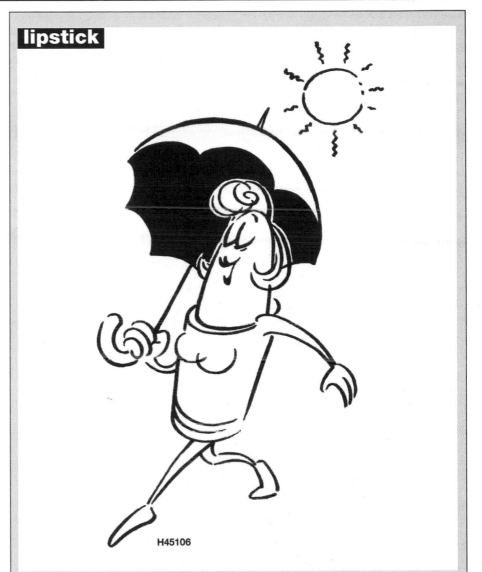

lipstick

H45106

A suntan is a burn! And every time you burn, you age – that's enough to make me go for the pale English Rose look, thanks!

alcohol. Meat eaters actually smell different from vegetarians.

2 Sweat is a mixture of water, salts and a little protein. It is produced by the skin's sweat glands which are found all over the body but tend to be more concentrated in areas like the hands. Although the skin is a major detoxifying organ the production of sweat is mainly part of temperature control. Dogs do not sweat and instead use air passing over their tongue which tend to be very large as a consequence. The evaporation of the water has a dramatic cooling effect especially if there is free movement of air

over the skin. Clothes, especially those with enclosed spaces act as 'double glazing' trapping air heated by the body. Sweat evaporation is also prevented which is why totally impervious material like plastic produces dampness. Very large amounts of body water can be lost in high temperatures or during a fever which must be replaced as the body cannot withstand dehydration for more than a day or so.

Symptoms

3 Profuse sweating can be embarrassing but rarely dangerous unless there is also significant

2

dehydration. Lack of sweating can cause overheating.

Causes

4 The main cause is a high environmental temperature but it can also occur with a fever. It is important to reduce the amount of clothes to allow this sweat to evaporate and cool the body as the brain in particular cannot tolerate high temperatures. A fan can help cool someone that much quicker. Inappropriate sweating can occur from alcohol abuse and anxiety. The smell of underarm sweat comes from bacteria which like warm damp environments not from the sweat itself which has little or no smell.

Prevention

5 Sweaty hands can be an embarrassment. Rinsing them in a dilute solution of aluminium chloride (from your pharmacist) will stop sweating for many hours. Many so-called deodorants simply mask the smell and do not stop sweating. It is possible to have a surgical block on the nerves which stimulate the sweat glands. This is a last resort.

Complications

6 Dehydration causes confusion, exhaustion and heart failure. Chronic dehydration can also damage the kidneys.

26 Warts & verrucas

1 Warts are common. Around 5% (1 in 20) school children will suffer from warts or verrucas. They are without doubt unsightly but actually quite harmless. They as also far less infectious than we once thought. Even so the possible (and controversial) link with cancer of the cervix needs to be taken seriously, so warts on the penis should be treated as soon as possible. Similarly the possible link between vaginal warts and cervical cancer needs medical advice if they are present.

Symptoms

2 Warts can appear anywhere on the body but are most common on the hands and feet. They can also appear at the anus, vagina and penis.

Causes

3 'Dirty' skin is not a cause, nor is poor hygiene. The papilloma virus which causes general skin warts may be a different strain from that which cause genital warts.

Prevention

4 Wearing protective foot wear at public baths may decrease the risk of passing on or picking up the infection but the public perception of 'lightening infection' is far from the truth.

Complications

5 Warts are not dangerous. Although they are a 'tumour' (this simply means growth) there is no connection between warts and say, skin cancer. Verrucas, which are simply inverted warts from the pressure of the foot, may cause pain when walking and can extend over the whole of the sole of the foot in severe cases. Genital warts should be removed at a GUM (genito urinary medical) clinic.

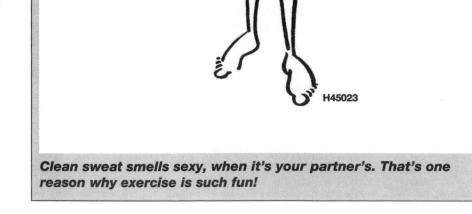

lipstick

H45023

Clean sweat smells sexy, when it's your partner's. That's one reason why exercise is such fun!

There is a controversial link with cervical cancer.

Self care

6 Warts appear to have a limited lifespan and eventually disappear on their own. It can be a frustrating wait as new warts may appear as the older warts depart. There are a number of wart removal creams available from the pharmacist. It takes great patience as repeated applications for more than a week are often required. Some GP practices offer a wart removal service.

27 Weight loss

1 Losing weight, or at least trying to lose weight, is very popular at the moment. This is perfectly reasonable if overweight, but there should be a good reason for the pounds dropping off. A significant loss of weight for no good reason (over 4.5 kg / 10 lb in 10 weeks without dieting or trying to lose weight) is not normal. Increasing exercise will decrease weight so long as calorie intake remains the same. Cutting down on alcohol is a good way to trim the waistline, but mysterious weight loss can result from certain medical conditions.

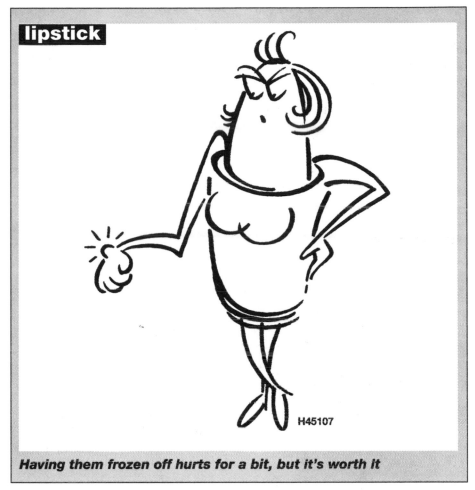

lipstick

H45107

Having them frozen off hurts for a bit, but it's worth it

2

Chapter 3
Air intake (breathing)

Contents

1 Asthma

1 Although deaths from asthma are on the decrease, for reasons we are not sure of, the number of people suffering from it is on the increase. Part of the problem may be pollution in our environment, particularly exhaust fumes. Some people blame double glazing and poor household ventilation although very cold countries have used double glazing for generations with no obvious problem. With around 2000 deaths each year in the UK, it should be taken very seriously. It can appear at any stage in life but is more common in younger people. Some people find the severity of the condition decreases as they get older. Thankfully modern treatments will prevent or stop the vast majority of asthma attacks.

Symptoms

2 The first sign of an attack can be as simple as a repeated cough which can rapidly develop into a frightening breathlessness and tightness in the chest. This is usually painless but after an attack there may be chest muscle strain which can ache. In the early stages a wheeze can be heard as the person breaths out. If they are suffering from a very serious attack there may be little or no wheeze or even the sound of breathing. They tend to sit up straight with their head slightly back with pursed lips. With severe attacks their lips may turn blue and they will be unable to speak. This is an emergency and you should dial 999/112.

Causes

3 Few medical conditions arouse such controversy when it comes to cause. Yes, some forms of asthma are triggered by things like pollen, hay or house dust but other forms seem to just happen with no apparent reason, although stress or a recent chest infection can act as triggers. People who have hay fever or other allergies in the family are most likely to develop asthma. Around 3% of adults suffer from the condition.

Prevention

4 There is as yet no way of preventing the condition but you can reduce the number and severity of attacks, particularly for someone with the allergic type of asthma. Keep a record of when and where they were with each attack. You may find it ties in with certain activities at work, the presence of a particular pet, the pollen count on that day or even what they had to eat. Some of these things cannot be changed but simple things like covering mattresses with a plastic cover to prevent dust mites or keeping certain flowers out of the house may make a difference. House dust mite faeces are a powerful trigger

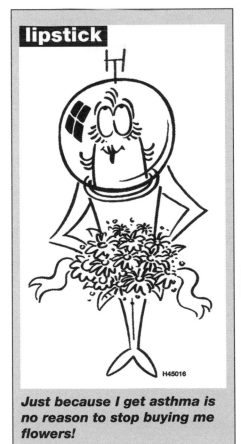

Just because I get asthma is no reason to stop buying me flowers!

3

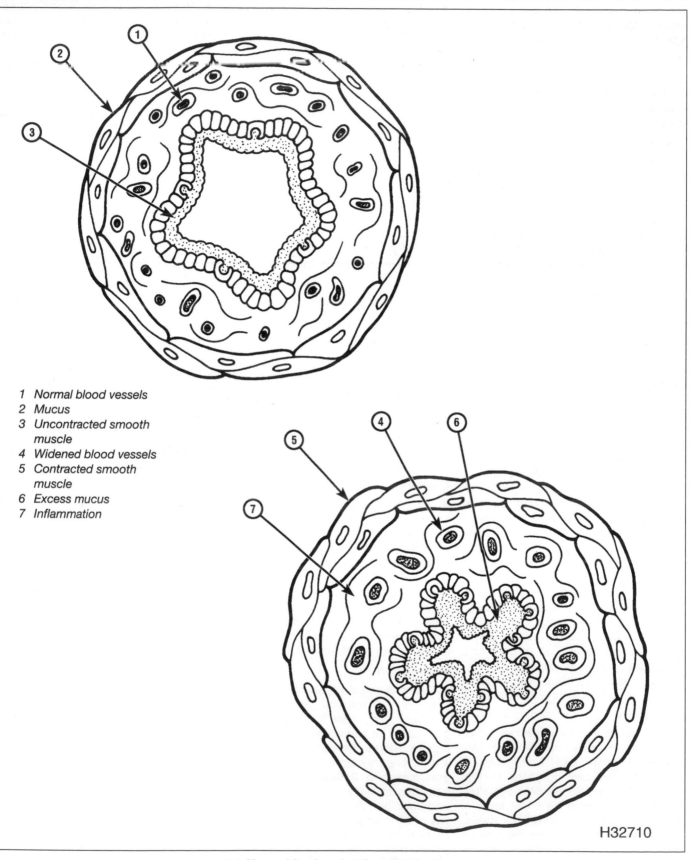

1 Normal blood vessels
2 Mucus
3 Uncontracted smooth
   muscle
4 Widened blood vessels
5 Contracted smooth
   muscle
6 Excess mucus
7 Inflammation

H32710

1.1 Normal (top) and asthmatic airways

for some asthma sufferers. Many vacuum cleaners can now be fitted with special filters which prevent this being blown into the air.

Complications

5 Badly controlled asthma can be dangerous especially if the symptoms are ignored.

Self care

6 General good health is important as is regular activity. Using an inhaler before physical activity can help reduce the risk of an attack. Peak flow rates should be regularly checked and compared with previous records, especially of attacks. It may point out triggers. Preventative inhalers once prescribed must be used regularly, even when feeling fine at the time. Nebulisers are often supplied by the GP practice on a loan basis or from support groups. In an emergency away from such machines, cut the large round end off a plastic lemonade bottle and fire the inhaler into the open end while the person breathes through the top hole.

7 Staying calm is vital when dealing with someone suffering an asthma attack. Find their inhaler and help them use it, dial 999/112 if it is a serious attack, reassure them, give them nothing to drink, allow them to sit in any position they find most comfortable, do not force them to lie down. If there is a nebuliser available use it sooner rather than later.

2 Breathlessness

1 Being breathless can be perfectly normal and is a natural response to the bodily system that detects that the oxygen in the blood has dropped. Large neck arties (carotid arteries) have small clumps of cells called the carotid bodies. These are sensitive to the levels of oxygen in the blood passing upwards from the heart. If this blood is even slightly low in oxygen the carotid bodies will send messages, along nerves, to the vital respiratory centres in the brain which in turn stimulates an increase in the depth and rate of breathing.

2 Excessive breathlessness from unfitness due to inadequate exercise is probably the commonest form of 'abnormal' breathlessness.

3 Almost any heart disorder can cause abnormal breathlessness. Atherosclerosis is a common disease of arteries that can lead to heart attacks, heart failure, strokes and other severe disorders.

4 Women who are seriously unfit at a time in life when they ought to be fit are in some danger of developing diseases that will cause a much more serious form of breathlessness than ordinary puffing on the second flight of stairs.

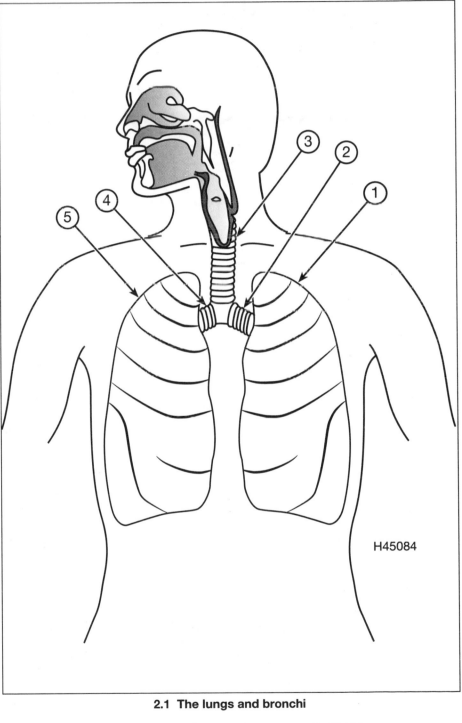

H45084

2.1 The lungs and bronchi

1 *Left lung*	3 *trachea*	5 *Right lung*
2 *Left bronchus*	4 *Right bronchus*	

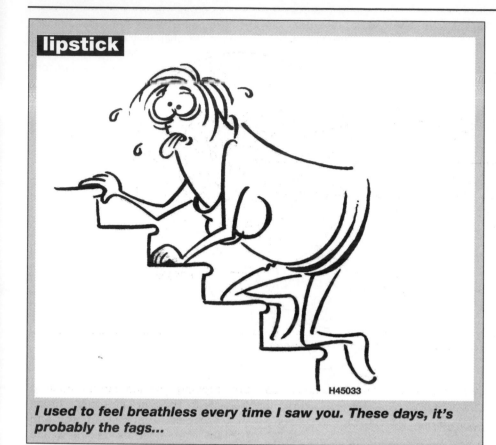

I used to feel breathless every time I saw you. These days, it's probably the fags...

Symptoms

5 Breathlessness after only moderate exertion means either being unfit or unwell.

Causes

6 Simply getting fit will work, as can losing weight, but breathlessness is also sometimes an important sign of disease. Conditions that will always cause breathlessness for this reason include:

· Spasm of the bronchial tubes (asthma).
· Collapse of the lung due to air between the lung and the chest wall (pneumothorax).
· Acute bronchitis.
· Chronic bronchitis.
· A breakdown of the air sacs so that the area of tissue available for oxygen passage is much reduced (emphysema).

7 Along with a lot of other medical problems, smoking is a particularly important cause of breathlessness and does this in several ways. Cigarette smoke contains carbon monoxide, a poisonous gas that combines so tightly with haemoglobin in the blood that the affected haemoglobin can't perform its normal function of transporting oxygen around the body. It is also a major factor for atherosclerosis.

8 So called 'panic reactions' can cause very rapid breathing without actual breathlessness generally brought on through over anxiety. If this is persisted in for a time so much carbon dioxide is breathed out that the blood becomes alkaline and the calcium levels drop. A strange tingling numbness creeps into the hands and feet making the person even more anxious thus creating a vicious circle.

Diagnosis

9 Any abnormal breathlessness, other than from being overweight or unfit needs a doctor's attention and should not be ignored.

3 Bronchitis

1 Far from being simple bags or balloons, the lungs are complex structures with strong tubes to bring large quantities of air into and out of the lungs, delicate thin linings for oxygen to pass through into the blood stream and carbon dioxide to leave it. Chemical irritants such as cigarette smoke or other environmental or industrial pollutants damage the ciliated cells which line the airways and help keep the lungs clean.

2 Coughing clears this gunge. When coughing up sputum takes place on most days, for at least three months of each year, usually in the winter months, the person has chronic bronchitis. Not surprisingly heavy smokers have chronic bronchitis, but refer to it simply as 'a smoker's cough'.

3 Although chronic bronchitis is a comparatively mild disease in the early stages with time and continued exposure to irritants, it is likely to progress to the condition called chronic obstructive pulmonary disease (COPD), in which large numbers of the tiny lung air sacs break down to form a smaller number of larger air spaces.

4 Smoking is especially dangerous in people with a persistent, productive cough. Chronic bronchitis and other forms of COPD affects around 10 per cent of female smokers.

Symptoms

5 In acute bronchitis there is a cough, at first dry but later with sputum, maybe fever for a few days, breathlessness and wheezing. There may be some pain in the chest. Occasionally a little blood may be coughed up. Any blood must be reported to a doctor even with a persistent cough.

Causes

6 Acute bronchitis in a previously healthy person is usually due to infection with a virus. In cigarette smokers this is often followed by other infections making matters worse. Industrial atmospheric pollution may also be a cause but most experts are convinced that by far the most important factor in the causation of serious bronchitis is cigarette smoking.

Diagnosis

7 A doctor will recognise bronchitis through its characteristic sound through a stethoscope.

8 The patient may be asked to blow into a machine to check something called peak expiratory flow

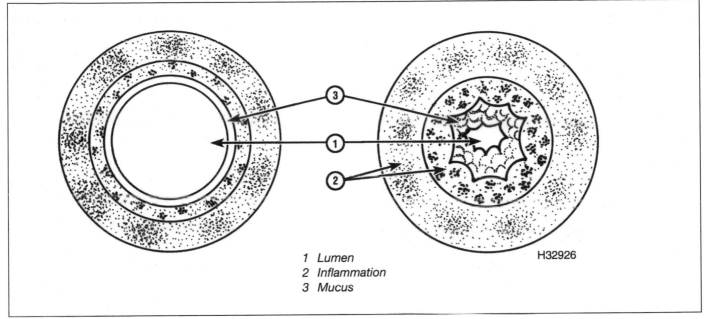

1 Lumen
2 Inflammation
3 Mucus

H32926

3.1 Normal (left) and inflamed bronchi

measurement. In a normal person asked to breathe out as forcibly as possible through the mouth, the rate of flow of the air rises rapidly to a peak and then declines steadily to zero. A normal person can breathe out at a peak rate of up to 8 litres a second, but In certain lung diseases, such as bronchitis, because of narrowing or partial obstruction of the bronchial tubes, the figure is much lower.

Prevention

9 Smoking is the main cause, but keeping the house free of smoke is also important.

Complications

10 It can cause the heart to enlarge and eventually be unable to pump the blood through the lungs. A heart and lung transplant is the only definitive treatment although drugs can help to an extent.

Treatment

11 Acute bronchitis is treated with antibiotics and usually responds well. There is no cure for chronic bronchitis, but stopping smoking can do much to alleviate it. There are now many drugs that can help relieve symptoms and perhaps even slow the decline of the lungs. Pulmonary rehabilitation can also help people live better lives with COPD.

4 Lung cancer

See Chapter 7.

3

NOTES

Chapter 4
Fuel & exhaust (digestion, blood & urogenital)

Contents

1 Anaemia

1 Perhaps the single greatest symptom of anaemia, which can be due to a lack of iron, is general tiredness. Red blood cells which transport oxygen around the body need iron to hold onto the oxygen until reaching those places needing it. A complex protein called haemoglobin binds the iron. Normally the body balances the amount of iron lost through periods or turnover of the blood cells with the amount taken in with the diet. If there is too much blood loss or not enough iron eaten she will become anaemic. Young women can outstrip their iron supply particularly during the growth spurt around puberty. Older women with poor diets can also suffer from anaemia, and this may be overlooked and their tiredness and confusion put down to age. The good news is that when recognised early it can often be treated quite easily.

Symptoms

• Skin, lips, tongue, nail beds or the inside of eyelids can be pale in colour although this doesn't really happen until the iron stores are quite low.
• Tiredness and weakness.
• Dizziness or fainting spells.
• Breathlessness, particularly following exercise.
• Fast heartbeat often felt in the neck or chest as palpitations.

Causes

2 The usual cause of anaemia is lack of iron or vitamin B12 in the diet. It can also arise following blood loss (eg, frequent nose bleeds). Conditions such as coeliac disease, some kidney problems and rheumatoid arthritis increase her risk of anaemia. Pregnancy places a greater demand on iron stores as there is an increase in the number of red blood cells to sustain oxygen supplies to the baby and form the baby's own haemoglobin.

3 Bleeding into the bowel will cause anaemia so it should be checked out immediately. There may be changes in the appearance of the motions, usually a black tar-like substance and there may be a weight loss for no apparent reason.

Prevention

4 A balanced diet will usually supply all the minerals needed. Young people going through their growth spurt need to make sure they are eating enough bread and other iron containing foods. Meat is a major source of iron so vegetarians may need extra iron containing foods although there is not always a need for iron supplements.

Complications

5 Relatively few people will die from anaemia but it can cause accidents through tiredness and lower her defence against minor illness. It also makes hearts work harder, not a good idea if there is already a cardiac problem. Strangely it can cause a 'spooning' of the fingernails (a drop of water can be held in the nail) which is one of the ways that doctors recognise the condition.

4

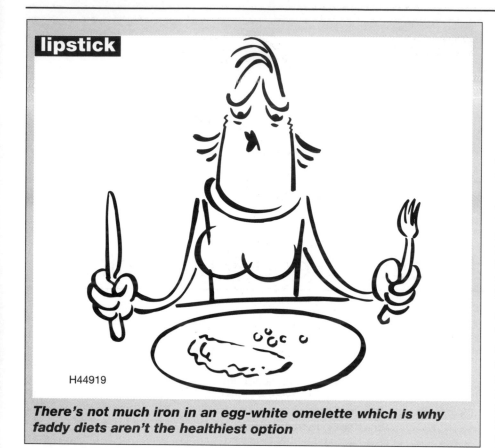

lipstick

H44919

There's not much iron in an egg-white omelette which is why faddy diets aren't the healthiest option

Self care

6 If you suspect anaemia and there is no obvious reason for it, do not suggest iron supplements until blood tests are performed and the doctor advised. Taking iron before the test makes it difficult to tell the cause of anaemia in the first place.

7 If anaemia is confirmed by a blood test, the doctor may prescribe iron tablets, injections or, occasionally, vitamin B12 injections. You can also help by making sure there are plenty of iron-rich foods, such as red meat, wholemeal bread, dried fruit and leafy vegetables to eat.

2 Angina (angina pectoris)

1 Acute angina is a pain not a compliment. It is more common in men. Angina is a symptom of the artery disease atherosclerosis which affects many arteries in the body, causing narrowing and partial obstruction to the blood flow. In this case, the arteries

concerned are the coronary arteries of the heart. These arteries and their branches supply the very actively moving heart muscle with the blood it needs to keep beating.

2 If the coronary arteries have been narrowed and can't get the blood to the heart muscle fast enough to meet the demand, abnormal levels of substances such as lactic acid collect in the muscle to the point of causing pain. This pain is angina.

Symptoms

3 The pain usually comes on after a certain amount of exertion, such as walking a particular distance or climbing a certain number of stairs.

4 It may be of very variable severity, even in the same person, and may be affected by factors such as cold weather, a change of temperature as when going outside from a warm house, the strength of the wind, the state of mind, and the length of time since the last meal. One of the things that can most readily bring on an attack is to try to walk against a strong cold wind.

5 The pain may be so mild as to be

hardly a pain – more a feeling of uneasiness or pressure in the chest – or so severe as to stop any further activity. It is often linked with breathlessness and belching. Simply stopping activity can make the angina soon settle. It is quite common for angina to remain at a fairly constant level of severity for years thus: 'stable angina'.

6 Unstable angina is a severe and dangerous form of angina. Pain becomes more frequent and prolonged, and may occur at rest. The accurate predictability of pain onset in terms of its relation to a given amount of exertion is lost, and the risk of a heart attack is increased. Trying to 'walk through the pain barrier' is life-threatening and immediate rest is vital.

Causes

7 Narrowing and hardening of the coronary arteries limits the rate blood can get to the heart muscle, in spite of its needs. When a coronary artery or a branch is reduced in bore by more than 50 per cent a rise in demand cannot be fully met and angina is a certain consequence.

8 A similar pain can be experienced elsewhere in the body under conditions of inadequate blood supply. If the main artery to the leg, for instance, is narrowed by atherosclerosis, pain occurs in the calf after walking a certain distance (claudication).

Diagnosis

9 An electrocardiograph (ECG), taken during exercise (a 'treadmill test') shows a characteristic pattern. It can be difficult telling the difference between angina and a heart attack so any chest pain which settles on rest must be reported to the doctor. Similarly if the pain refuses to settle even with rest. The pain from a heart attack often radiates up into the jaw, through to the back and down the left arm.

10 The principal difference between this pain and the pain of angina is in its duration. Anginal pain will nearly always stop when the factor that has brought it on – exertion, stress, emotion, etc – ceases. But the pain of a heart attack is the pain of an area of heart muscles that is being damaged by deprivation of blood, and may last for hours.

11 Obviously most chest pain is neither

angina or a heart attack but rather indigestion, rib muscle pain or cramp from sitting crouched over for too long.

12 Because angina is more common in men, many women ignore symptoms, thinking 'it must be something I ate'. If a women you know gets pain and it seems to fit Dr Ian's description, persuade her to see a doctor.

Prevention

13 Not blocking up the coronary arteries in the first place is the name of the game. Once diagnosed and understood, angina can be prevented by keeping within the exertional limits that trigger it.

Treatment

14 'Nitrates' are the mainstay of treatment as they act very quickly to open up the arteries. The most common is glyceryl trinitrate (GTN), highly effective in controlling the pain of angina. The oral preparation may be taken in a tablet that is allowed to dissolve under the tongue and the pain is usually relieved in two to three minutes. The drug is also available in patches to be applied to the skin (transdermal patches) and sprays for under the tongue.

15 Women may be taking anti-impotence drugs, as there is some evidence they improve sexual arousal but as for men these react badly with nitrate causing a, sometimes serious, drop in blood pressure.

16 Surgery can be used to open up the blocked arties. An effective treatment for angina is to have your narrowed coronary arteries widened by a procedure called coronary angioplasty. This is done using a thin tube called a balloon catheter. This has a sausage-shaped balloon segment near one end and it is pushed into the narrowed part of the artery. The balloon is then inflated to distend the constriction.

17 The alternative to angioplasty, coronary artery bypass, now carries very little risk and the results are excellent. Segments of vein are used to provide a new channel by which the blood can be shunted past the blocked part of the artery. Many surgeons prefer to connect a local artery from the chest wall, a mammary artery, to the narrowed coronary beyond the point of the block.

18 The most recent advances in methods of re-opening narrowed

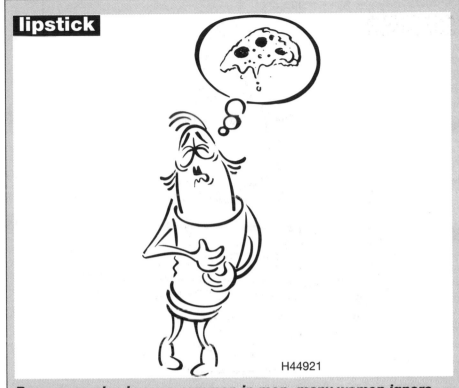

lipstick

H44921

Because angina is more common in men, many women ignore symptoms, thinking 'it must be something I ate'

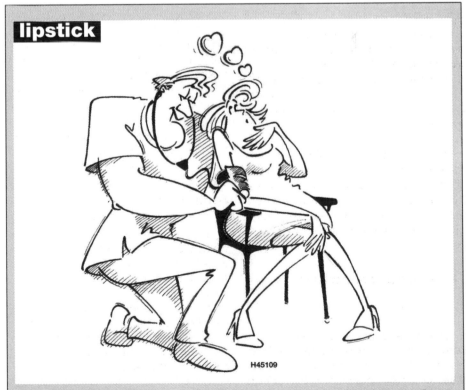

lipstick

H45109

Anti-impotence drugs can improve sexual arousal but sometimes also cause a serious drop in blood pressure

4

coronary arteries include the use of catheters with high-speed rotating cylindrical cutters that shave away the atheromatous plaques and suck out the debris. There are also catheter cutters that pulverize plaques into fragments so small that they can be safely carried away by the bloodstream.

3 Atrial fibrillation

1 Any change in the regularity of heart beat can be frightening but most are harmless or easily treatable. Anxiety, exhaustion, alcohol and even too much tea or coffee can make the heart skip beats. The control of the heart beat starts with a small clump of special muscle called the sinoatrial node. This is the natural pacemaker of the heart. Its impulses are conveyed from there to another node at the junction between the upper and the lower chambers, called the atrioventricular node.

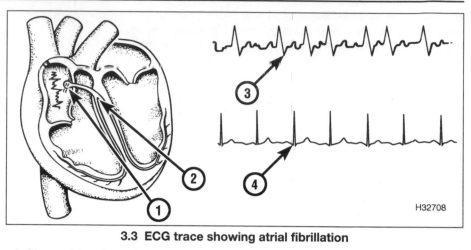

3.3 ECG trace showing atrial fibrillation

1 Sino-atrial node   2 AV node   3 Irregular heart beat   4 Normal heart beat

2 It is the atrioventricular node that determines the rate of contraction of the lower chambers, the ventricles, and thus the pulse rate.

3 Atrial fibrillation is a condition in which the upper chambers of the heart contracts at a very high rate and in an erratic manner. The result is an irregular beating of the ventricles, because the atrioventricular node receives more electrical impulses than it can conduct.

4 Atrial fibrillation increases with age, so suffers are as follows:
• Women aged 65 to 74 years: 2.4 per cent.
• Women aged 75 years and older: 5.6 per cent.

5 People who already have heart disease are particularly vulnerable and men tend to suffer more often than women.

Symptoms

6 Atrial fibrillation is a completely irregular, but usually fast, heart beat rate. It is often in excess of 140 beats per minute, but the rate may be anywhere between 50-200 beats per minute. In the early stages, symptoms seem more prominent and affected people are usually unpleasantly aware of the irregularity of the heart's action.

Causes

7 Atrial fibrillation may be due to overactivity of the thyroid gland, anaemia, excessive alcohol intake or inflammation of the heart muscle, but simple things like excess coffee or tea drinking can trigger it too. Athletes can suffer from it when they push themselves too far. Some heart conditions can also make it more likely.

Diagnosis

8 Comparing the rate of heart beat by stethoscope and the pulse at the wrist is a simple test.

9 One of the most important tests is the electrocardiograph (ECG).

10 Blood tests can also be useful in the

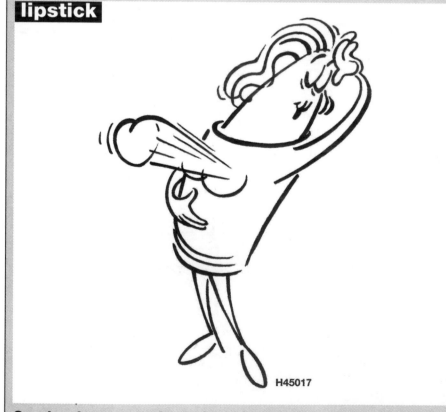

lipstick

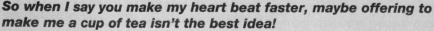

So when I say you make my heart beat faster, maybe offering to make me a cup of tea isn't the best idea!

diagnosis. They may show anaemia, which may be complicating the situation, impaired kidney function, thyroid gland overactivity (thyrotoxicosis).

Prevention

11 Regular checks on blood pressure and treatment for raised pressure can reduce the chances of developing the heart problems that cause atrial fibrillation.

Complications

12 The risk of stroke in people with atrial fibrillation is about twice that in the general population.

Treatment

13 The first step is to be sure whether the cause of the atrial fibrillation is known and can be treated. If so, this may be all the treatment that is required.

14 Digoxin, beta blockers or calcium channel blockers, or a combination of these drugs can help. Aspirin or warfarin may be prescribed to reduce the risk from blood clots.

15 Cardioversion (electric shock to the heart under general anaesthetic) is most likely to be successful.

4 Bladder cancer

See Chapter 7

5 Bowel cancer

See Chapter 7

6 Constipation

1 There is a fascination with our bodily function but none more than going to the toilet. Toilets in Germany even have a small shelf on to which the motions fall so that you can take a good look before flushing. Similarly, 'being regular' is ingrained into people from a young age with great consternation if the daily poo is not passed. In fact there is no 'normal' number of times you need to go to the toilet. What we do know is that putting it off for too long can cause constipation

and tears around the anus. Thankfully, the serious causes of constipation are relatively rare, particularly in people under 45 years old.

Symptoms

2 These are self evident yet vary between people. Simply not passing a motion in the morning with no other symptoms is considered by some to be 'constipation'. In truth it has to be a significant change in normal bowel movements with very irregular and difficult to pass motions before the label constipation can be used. There may also be abdominal pain and bloating.

Causes

3 It can range from simple (eg, lack of activity) to serious (eg, blockage of the bowel from cancer). Advanced age, compounded with a disability can be the big factors for reduced activity and subsequent constipation. Also not drinking enough non-alcoholic fluids and a lack of fibre in the diet are major

factors. Paradoxically, overuse of laxatives can also cause a severe constipation, particularly once they are stopped. Some medicines, particularly pain killers containing codeine, are powerful constipating agents. Stress or 'holding on' can cause constipation and this is made worse by a poor diet.

Prevention

4 Most of the preventative measures are just sensible attention to the things that cause constipation such as:
- Drink more, particularly pure fruit juices.
- Take more activity.
- Avoid laxatives (do not stop suddenly, gradually reduce them).
- Eat more fibre and fruit.
- Check any medicines with the pharmacist.

Complications

5 Thankfully, constipation itself is very rarely harmful even though it can be very uncomfortable, even painful. The big

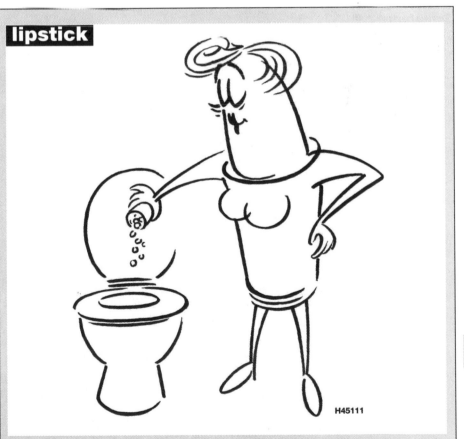

lipstick

Laxatives? No thanks – hand me another Bucks fizz. My doctor says fruit juice and plenty of it is good for you!

danger is ignoring the warning signs of something more serious and not having it checked out soon enough, as bowel cancer can be cured when caught early.

6 Some symptoms need urgent medical attention:

• Vomiting after a few days total constipation.
• Severe abdominal pain.
• Any blood or black tar-like material in the motion.
• Unexplained weight loss.
• A sudden unexplained change in bowel habit.

7 Cystitis

1 As almost all cystitis is linked to a bacterium found in the bowel (E Coli) it may be the closer proximity of the anus to the vagina which makes women suffer most from this infection of the bladder. This may give some clues as to how to avoid it in the first place.

Symptoms

• Burning sensation when passing water.

• A feeling of needing to pass water very often and not quite emptying the bladder each time.
• Crampy pains in the lower abdomen just above the pubis.

Causes

2 E coli bacteria are the single greatest cause but it also appears to happen spontaneously with some women suffering more than others. Any reduction in the body's ability to fight infection such diabetes and the use of steroids for chronic conditions like rheumatoid arthritis tend to make infection more common. Kidney stones and reflux (where the urine can pass back from the bladder toward the kidney) can also increase the frequency of infection.

3 So-called honeymoon cystitis is associated with vigorous and/or frequent sexual activity. In fact it is usually urethritis, an inflammation of the urethra (the tube through which urine leaves the bladder) - though the symptoms are very similar.

Prevention

4 Dehydration and a slow flow through the kidneys and bladder seem to make things worse, so drinking plenty of non-alcoholic fluids helps prevent cystitis in

the first place, cranberry juice which is slightly acidic is said to help prevent and treat cystitis. Wiping from the front to the back and using a fresh piece of toilet paper each time when finishing on the toilet may also help

5 Because it hurts to go, there's a temptation to drink less and hold on. Encourage her to drink plenty as this flushes out the infection and speeds up treatment.

Complications

6 It is rare for cystitis to go on to produce any serious harm and often disappears without any specific treatment unless there is an underlying cause. Repeated infections need to be reported to the doctor.

Self care

• A hot water bottle against the tummy eases the pain.
• Slightly acid drinks such as cranberry juice, lemon squash or pure orange juice change the urine so that bacteria cannot survive in it.
• Potassium citrate mixtures available from the pharmacist taste dreadful but can work wonders for some women.
• Carry and use wet wipes and always wipe front to back.

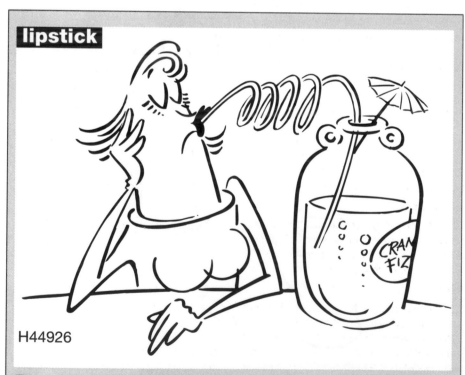

Encourage her to drink plenty as this flushes out the infection and speeds up treatment

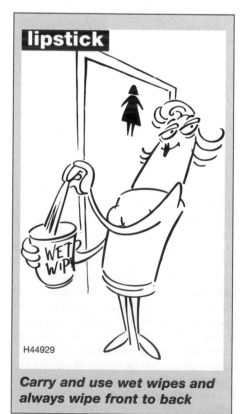

Carry and use wet wipes and always wipe front to back

Medical advice should be sought:

• If the infection is lasting more than a few days and/or there is also severe pain and/or a fever.
• If there is any blood or clots in the urine.
• If she is pregnant.
• If she is diabetic or taking steroids.

7 Take a urine sample from her first visit to the toilet in the morning. Tell her to pass the container swiftly through the stream just after she has started and use a clean, well-rinsed bottle. Special containers are available from the GP surgery.

8 Diabetes (mellitus)

1 There are two main types of diabetes, which is basically an inability of the body to control the level of sugar (glucose) in the blood stream.
2 Type I or insulin-dependency diabetes, in which the person produces little or no insulin, affects about one per cent of the population.
3 Type II diabetes, often called maturity-onset diabetes, is usually associated with obesity and can be regarded as a condition in which the body cells don't react to insulin, or in which the amount of insulin produced by the pancreas – and this may be near normal – is not enough for the excessive tissue bulk.
4 Type II diabetes can often be treated simply by dieting and weight loss (see *Obesity*). This reduces the sugar demands but, possibly more important, it also makes lowered demands on the insulin supply. Other cases require oral anti-diabetic drugs which stimulate the pancreas to produce more insulin, and some people with this type of diabetes also require injections of insulin.
5 Sugar in the blood can only vary between certain fairly narrow limits if damage is to be avoided. A shortage of insulin as in diabetes, tends to cause the blood sugar levels to rise and an excessive rise is associated with the over-production of dangerous acidic substances called ketones.
6 There are around 1 million undiagnosed diabetic people in the UK and the number of people known to be affected is approaching 5% of the population. Fortunately the outlook is getting better with the increasing possibility of a cure rather than treatment and with much better understanding of how to minimise the complications of diabetes.

Symptoms

7 Thirst, excessive urine and, in Type I diabetes, weight loss and tiredness are the major symptoms.

Causes

8 Diabetes either results from the failure of the specialised pancreas cells called islet cells to produce the hormone insulin or the cells of the body not being able to respond correctly to insulin. This hormone is essential for the building up of important large molecules, such as fats, proteins and glycogen from small molecules such as glucose and amino acids, and for the uptake of glucose for energy by cells such as muscle cells.
9 The cause of the damage to the islet cells of the pancreas is an auto-immune disorder, probably related to a virus infection which somehow alters pancreas tissue so as to render it unrecognisable as 'self' to the immune system. The lack of sensitivity of cells to insulin is almost always caused by obesity.
10 Diabetes in pregnancy is well known and can disappear after the baby is born. Conversely, the severity of maternal diabetes is often reduced during pregnancy as the baby's own pancreas helps to control maternal blood glucose levels. Unfortunately this protection is lost when the baby is born. It can also cause babies to be very large at birth.

Diagnosis

11 Diabetes is diagnosed by testing for sugar in the urine, and by checking the levels of blood sugar particularly at different times of the day.

Prevention

12 There is reason for optimism that the immune system process that causes Type I diabetes in future can be prevented and that if it is recognized early enough and blocked, the disease can be prevented. The risk of Type II diabetes can be almost eliminated through avoiding obesity.

Complications

13 Hypoglycaemia is an abnormally low level of sugar (glucose) in the blood. This is a dangerous state as the brain is totally dependent on a constant supply of glucose as fuel. Hypoglycaemia occurs when there is a failure of balance between insulin dosage, food intake and energy expenditure.
14 Unfortunately, hypoglycaemia is often mistaken for drunkenness as the person can be forgetful, unsteady and have slurred speech. The commonest cause of a 'hypo', as this condition is known by diabetics, is not quite matching the amount of food against the amount of insulin injected. Skipping breakfast is a typical example although increased exercise can also mean that glucose is used up faster than normal causing a drop in blood sugar levels.
15 Insulin dependent diabetics should always carry readily digested sugar but also take a biscuit or some other complex carbohydrate which takes longer to digest to prevent a sudden relapse. The drop in blood sugar can also be caused by overdosage with oral hypoglycaemic drugs, especially chlorpropamide.

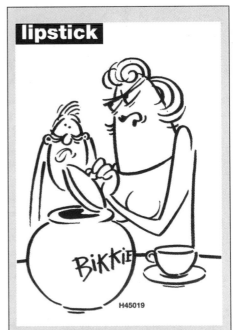

lipstick

BiKKiE

H45019

It's a good excuse to explain why you came home in a state and ate all the biscuits but I'm not buying it!

4

16 Glucagon is a protein hormone produced by the islet cells of the pancreas, which has an effect opposite to that of insulin. By causing glycogen, stored in the liver, to break down to glucose, it increases the amount of sugar in the bloodstream. In an emergency glucagon can be given by injection and many diabetic people carry a small case with instructions. This can be life saving when given and can cause little harm if given for the wrong reasons so long as the person is seen by a doctor.

17 Poorly controlled diabetes can lead to a wide range of long-term complications, including eye, kidney, circulatory and heart problems.

Treatment

18 Type I diabetes is treated with insulin injections, and diet and exercise control, all monitored by frequent checks of the blood sugar levels. Pancreatic or islet cell transplantation is still experimental but there have been major advances.

19 Type II diabetes is treated by weight loss, diet control, oral hypoglycaemic drugs and if necessary insulin injections.

9 Heart attack

1 Heart muscle must have a continuous supply of oxygen and energy. It gets this from arteries which only supply the cardiac muscle and a small amount from the blood inside the heart itself. An acute myocardial infarction (heart attack) is what happens when the blood supply to a part of the heart muscle has been cut off by blockage of one of the coronary arteries. When blood is suddenly cut off the muscle starts to die. About five people in every 1000, mostly men, suffer a myocardial infarction in the UK each year and although women have a lower rate in their younger age this rises to meet the rate in older men.

Symptoms

2 Not all or any of these symptoms can happen but they are the commonest indicators:

- Crushing central chest pain.
- Breathlessness.
- Clammy, sweat and grey complexion.
- Dizziness, sickness and vomiting.
- Restlessness.

3 The pain often travels (radiates) to the neck, jaws, ears, arms and wrists. Less often, it travels to between the shoulder blades or to the abdomen. The pain does not pass on resting as in angina (see *Angina*).

4 Severe pain is not always present. In less major cases pain may be absent and there is evidence that up to 20 per cent of mild heart attacks are not recognised as such, or even as significant illness by those affected. Many women who might have been saved have died because they did not recognise or believe that they were suffering from a heart attack.

Causes

5 The cause of a heart attack is the blockage caused by a clot (thrombosis) from a plaque of atherosclerosis. Blockage of a branch of a coronary artery occurs when blood, which will not normally clot within the circulation, is prompted to do so by a roughened plaque of fatty, degenerative, cholesterol-containing material called atheroma in the inner lining of the vessel.

6 When total blockage occurs, part of the heart muscle loses its blood supply (myocardial infarction) and dies. Depending on the size of the artery blocked, this dead area may involve the full thickness of the heart wall, or only part. The heart cannot continue to function as a pump if more than a certain proportion of the muscle is destroyed.

Risk factors include:

- Smoking.
- Being overweight.
- High blood pressure.
- High blood cholesterol level.
- A diet high in saturated fats (animal fats).
- Diabetes.
- A family history of heart disease.
- Lack of regular exercise.
- Occupation (especially if sedentary and stressful).

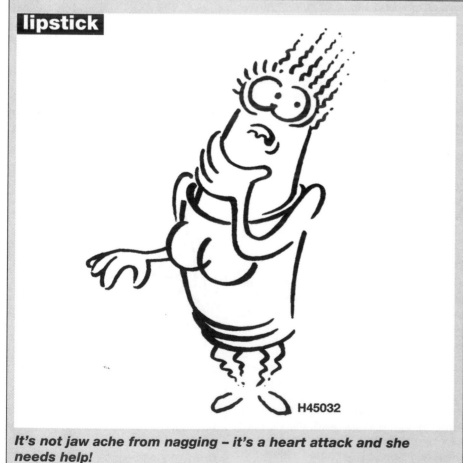

lipstick

H45032

It's not jaw ache from nagging – it's a heart attack and she needs help!

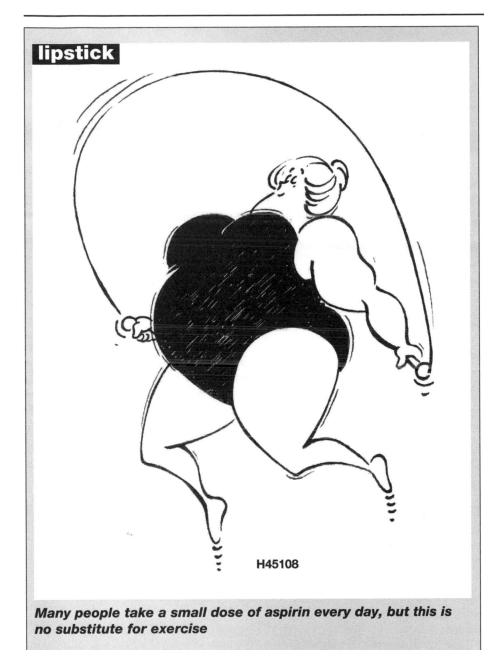

lipstick

H45108

Many people take a small dose of aspirin every day, but this is no substitute for exercise

Diagnosis

7 Although an ECG (electro-cardiograph), much loved by TV soap dramas, can show which part of the heart muscle has been damaged it is by no means a certain test for a heart attack and it requires a health professional's judgment which may be that treatment is required irrespective of the ECG result.

8 A blood test will look for certain heart muscle proteins that are only found in high levels immediately after a heart attack. These are also useful in confirming the diagnosis.

Prevention

• Your diet should include a high proportion of fruit and fresh vegetables.

• A Mediterranean diet with emphasis on olive oil rather than butter is desirable.

• Moderate alcohol intake – such as one glass of wine a day – may be helpful.

• Stop smoking permanently, increase exercise if sedentary and avoid saturated fats.

• Many people take a small dose of aspirin every day as a routine precaution, but this is no substitute for exercise, stopping smoking and avoiding saturated animal fats.

Complications

9 There are certain complications which can happen soon after a heart attack while some only appear weeks or maybe months later. Immediate complications are:

• Dangerous irregular heart rhythms and very fast or very slow rates.

• Dangerous drops in blood pressure.

• Fluid build-up in and around the lungs.

• Clots forming in the deep veins of the legs or pelvis (deep vein thrombosis).

• Rupture of the heart wall.

10 Later complications are:

• Ballooning (aneurysm) of the damaged heart wall, which becomes thin and weak.

• Increased risk of another heart attack in the future.

• Angina.

• Poor heart action causing breathlessness and build-up of fluid in the ankles and legs (oedema).

• Depression, loss of confidence, loss of sex drive, and fear of having sex which is common and unfounded.

Treatment

11 Thanks to the efforts of organisations such as the Red Cross, Knights of Malta and St John Ambulance many lives have been saved by timely and efficient first aid. If the affected person is not breathing and has no pulse, immediate lifesaving treatment with cardiopulmonary resuscitation (CPR) must be started (see *First Aid*). Dial 999 and call for an ambulance; tell the despatcher that it is for a heart attack.

12 Clot-dissolving injections are now routinely used in hospital. These can break down the clot in the coronary artery and allow the damaged heart muscle to recover, sometimes completely, but they must preferably be given within 24 hours of the heart attack happening. In an uncomplicated recovery it is normal to be home within a week or less. Work can be restarted 4-12 weeks after the attack, depending on the level of physical exertion involved with the job. Driving can restart after one month, but DVLA and the motor insurance company must be informed of the heart attack.

4

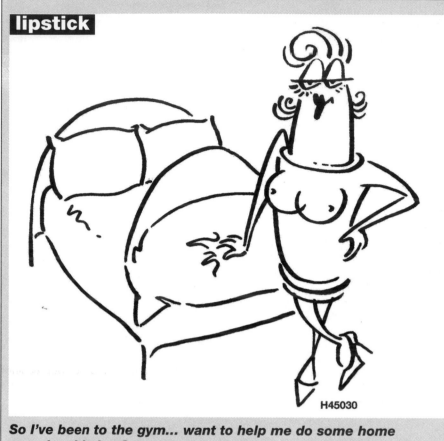

So I've been to the gym... want to help me do some home exercise, big boy?

13 Rather than avoiding any exercise it is now known that a return to normal levels of activity helps to prevent any further attacks and this includes sex.

10 Indigestion and heartburn

1 Indigestion is a vague term covering basically those things caused by stomach acid not being in the right place at the right time and is more common in middle-aged people, after heavy meals or alcohol consumption and is often worse at night. A new term, Gastro-Oesophageal-Reflux-Dysfunction (GORD) has take over as it is increasingly seen as a condition in its own right. Regurgitation or reflux of acid from the stomach into the oesophagus (gullet) is painful although rarely dangerous. Stomach acid escapes into the gullet causing chest pain and can be mistaken for a heart attack. Severe reflux can occur with a hiatus hernia.

Symptoms

• Vague pain below the ribcage extending into the throat.
• Acid taste in the mouth.
• Excessive wind.

Causes

• Classically after a heavy meal or drinking.
• Rich food, often with a high fat content.
• Excessive smoking.
• A leaking valve at the neck of the stomach (Hiatus hernia).

Prevention

• Avoid food which provokes an attack.
• Sleep with your upper body propped up with pillows.
• Avoid eating just before bed time.
• Eat small meals more often.
• Avoid aspirin and drugs like ibuprofen (non-steroidal anti-inflammatory drugs).

Complications

2 Most indigestion is harmless but annoying. The acid refluxing into the throat does not appear to cause any serious damage. The greatest danger is ignoring repeated attacks or confusing them with a heart attack. There is some evidence of a link between a relatively rare condition (Barrett's) where acid producing cells are found in the gullet instead of the stomach and oesophageal cancer.

Self care

• Pharmacists will advise about indigestion remedies (antacids).
• Avoid taking large amounts of sodium bicarbonate (baking soda) as this is turned into salt in the body.
• A glass of low fat milk before bed can help.

Treatment

3 As GORD becomes increasingly recognised as a condition in its own right many doctors advocate specific treatment using drugs which move the acid contents of the stomach more quickly into the next part of the gut, the duodenum. An alternative is H2 blockers which stop production of acid in the first place. Antacids have a limited effect and there is often a so called 'rebound' effect where more acid is produced once the antacid has been used up by stomach acid.

11 High blood pressure (hypertension)

1 Myths surround every aspect of blood pressure. It helps to know what is being measured in the first place. Blood pressure (BP) is always written as one number over another thus: 120/70. Neither of these numbers has anything to do with the person's age, height or weight. They are simply measurements of the heart's ability to overcome pressure from a cuff placed around the arm or leg and inflated.

2 As the cuff is slowly deflated, the sound of the blood pushing its way past is heard in a stethoscope placed over the artery. This is the maximum pressure reached by the heart during its contraction. As the pressure is further released the sound gradually muffles and disappears; the lowest pressure in the blood system. Putting the two pressures over each other gives a ratio of the blood pressure while the heart is contracting (systolic) over the pressure while the heart is refilling with blood ready for the next contraction (diastolic). The lower pressure actually represents the pressure caused by the major arteries contracting keeping the blood moving while the heart refills.

3   There is no 'normal' blood pressure as it constantly changes within the same person and depends on what they are doing at the time. A blood pressure of above 160/100 for anyone at rest should be investigated. A single reading of blood pressure is useless. At least three readings over a few weeks are required. Simply having blood pressure checked can make it rise in some people (called the white coat effect). Self-testing using machines from the pharmacist is a good idea.

Symptoms

4   Hypertension is called the silent killer for good reason. Most people do not realise that they are suffering from high blood pressure until something serious happens. As the pressure steadily rises, damage occurs to the arteries, kidney and heart. For this reason alone it is worth having a blood pressure check every year or so over the age of 45 years. Most women will have their BP check more often during child bearing age or when they are seeing their GP for HRT. There may be some warning signs such as blood in the urine or loss of vision right at the edges (tunnel vision) but these tend to come on after high blood pressure has been there for some time.

Causes

5   There are two types of hypertension. One is genetically linked and increases the risk for a lifestyle likely to cause hypertension. High salt intake, fatty food, obesity, stress, alcohol abuse and lack of activity all contribute to hypertension.

6   The second type is caused by some medical conditions which have an effect on blood pressure. Kidney problems are a good example.

Prevention

7   Taking a look at the causes of high blood pressure and prevention explains itself.
- Cutting down on salt.
- Reducing weight.
- Reducing fat intake.
- Drinking alcohol in moderation.

Staying active

8   Even 15 minutes each day of activity causing slight breathlessness is of all is perhaps the easiest prevention and has the most dramatic effect for decreasing the risk from hypertension.

Complications

9   Stroke and heart attacks are two of the most common complications from hypertension. It can also damage the kidneys and liver.

12 HIV & AIDS

1   Prejudice, misunderstanding and bigotry surround the endemic path of HIV in our society. Following infection with the Human Immunodeficiency Virus (HIV) there are less white blood cells called CD4 thus lowering the body's resistance to infection. At least 25 million people in the world are HIV positive. Although the virus only appeared in the UK in 1982 there are over 4,000 new cases reported each year with perhaps 10 times this number unrecognised and the number is increasing. Bad news but it is not a matter of doom and gloom. New treatments are significantly extending life expectancy. Even so, the name of the game is prevention.

Symptoms

2   Early stages of infection generally go unnoticed and it needs an antibody test

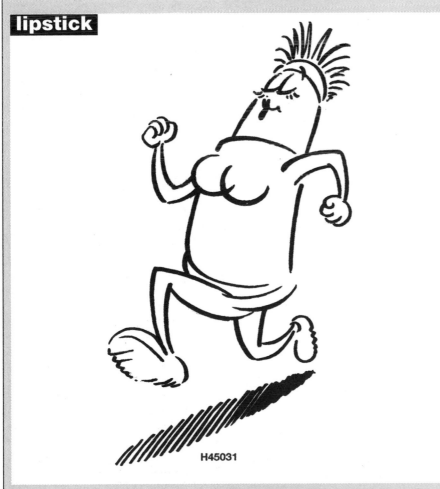

lipstick

H45031

Well, slight breathlessness is the right description of what it does to me, but 15 minutes? I should be so lucky! Maybe I should take up running!

4

from a blood or saliva sample to confirm the presence of the virus. The appearance of the antibodies can take months and is known as seroconversion. A vague non specific illness similar to flu or glandular fever sometimes follows the infection at around 6 to 7 weeks later. A variable period of time, years even, can then pass completely symptom free. The occurrence of oral thrush, persistent herpes (cold sores) or strange chest infections which clear only slowly with treatment are ominous signs of the body's declining ability to fight off other infections.

Causes

3 Body fluids are often cited as the carrier of the virus. Actually this can be narrowed down to blood, semen and saliva. Although the risk of infection from saliva is extremely small it makes sense to avoid obvious risks such as oral sex without adequate protection. Similarly, there are no cases of doctors passing on the virus to their patient, although a number of doctors suffer from infection in the opposite direction. The main routes of infection are:

• Sexual transmission via blood from small cuts either in the mouth (oral sex), vagina, anus or penis.

• Blood transfusion in countries with poor medical resources is still a risk and you can buy a travel kit from your GP.
• Sharing dirty needles or even razor blades.

Prevention

4 According to the World Health Organisation (WHO) up to 90 per cent of those people infected in the world contracted HIV through heterosexual sex of whatever form. Dental dams, male and female condoms particularly those containing the spermicide non-oxynol-9 give a high degree of protection. Use stronger condoms; these will protect both you and your partner.

5 Although extra lubrication is often required, do not use an oil-based lubricant such as petroleum jelly, baby oil, margarine or butter. They will damage the condom. There are water-based lubricants available. If you are not sure, ask the chemist, they sell thousands of them and will not be embarrassed to give advice.

Self care

6 Healthy diets are not quite the same when HIV positive. Reducing cholesterol and fat intake will reduce the chances of having an early heart attack at say 60 years. Commonsense will prevail over how useful this diet will be to an HIV-infected woman, depending upon her age on infection. In fact, full fat milk, cheeses, creamy yoghurt, butter and ice cream are all preferable to their low fat alternatives. Fat supplies not only a valuable energy source but also vitamins which are only found in fatty products. As better treatments come on stream this becomes less important and the other risks to health become more important.

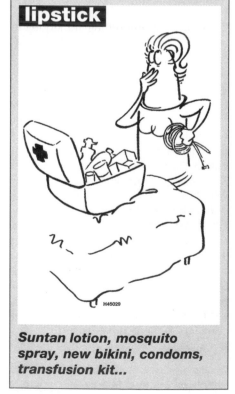

Suntan lotion, mosquito spray, new bikini, condoms, transfusion kit...

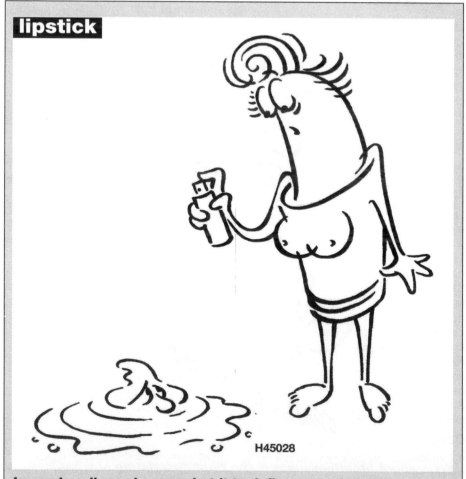

Lavender oil may be sexy, but it took five seconds from application to meltdown! We'll use the proper stuff in future

13 Kidney infections & stones

1 Without kidneys we would have steak and nothing pies. One of the great underrated organs, kidneys are more than just filters, they also control blood pressure and stimulate the production of red blood cells but their main role is to control the amount of fluid in the body and flush out toxins. If the body has too much water on board it becomes 'oedematous' and this can build up in the blood damaging vital organs such as the brain. If there is too little water the body becomes dehydrated which can also damage vital organs not least the kidney itself as it must pass a critical minimum of fluid to avoid damage.

2 There are usually two kidneys, one on each side just beneath the back rib cage. They are connected to the bladder by long tubes (ureters). Sometimes there can be two ureters coming from the one kidney. In most cases this will not cause any problems but it can sometimes make infections more likely to occur. Kidney infections are relatively rare but can be serous. Similarly, stones are common and can form in the kidney and block the ureter which not only cause pain but may also make infection more likely.

Symptoms

3 It is hard to miss a kidney infection as they can be extremely painful with a heavy dragging sensation in the back. A high temperature is common and there may be blood clots in the urine. Tenderness over the muscles of the back can also occur. Vomiting is common. Stones can form from calcium or oxalate (a form of acid) and can be a sign of a mineral imbalance in the blood. Renal colic is often described as the worst pain known to man or woman and often requires very powerful pain killers to control. The pain typically starts from the back but passes down to the groin. Small pieces of stone along with blood clots may be found in the urine.

Causes

4 Infections can occur for no apparent reason but are also associated with congenital malformations of the kidney (two or more ureters draining the kidney). Chronic dehydration is also a common

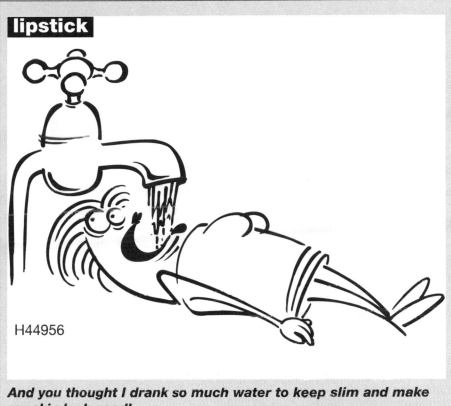

And you thought I drank so much water to keep slim and make my skin look good!

factor. Reflux where the urine is forced back up the ureter is also a factor as is the presence of a stone.

Prevention

5 Both infections and stones can be prevented by drinking plenty of plain water each day but there is often a familial connection.

Complications

6 Infections, dehydration and the back pressure from obstructions like stones can damage the kidney. If this happens repeatedly the kidney can cease to function and can disturb normal blood pressure and blood function such as anaemia.

Treatment

7 First line treatment with antibiotics will treat the infection although they do tend to recur if the underlying cause is not addressed. Stones can be removed by various methods such as ultrasound which disintegrates the stone. In some cases a long wire with a basket is used to pull the stone down the ureter. In very severe cases it may be necessary to

perform surgery and if the kidney has ceased to function it will need to be removed.

8 Fortunately the remaining kidney is more than capable of performing all the required tasks. If both kidneys have failed dialysis is required until a suitable donor kidney can be found. Thousands of lives are saved every year by people having the good sense to carry a donor card with them at all times.

14 Peptic ulcers

1 Treatment for peptic ulcers was once the single greatest cause of surgery. From a major operation with its own dangers to life, peptic ulcers are now treated with drugs with virtually no risk. These ulcers are found in two places, within the lining of the stomach (a gastric ulcer) and within the lining of the first part of the small intestine (a duodenal ulcer). Gastric ulcers are more common in people over 40 years although prolonged use of high doses of oral steroids, eg, for

4

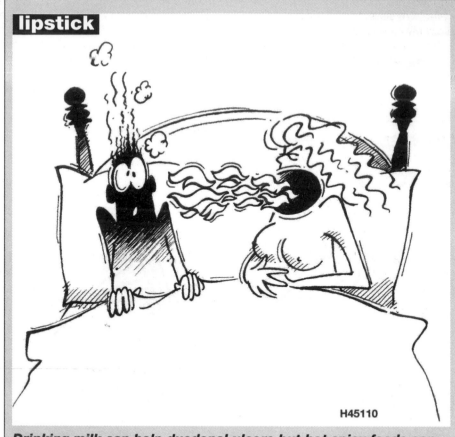

lipstick

H45110

Drinking milk can help duodenal ulcers but hot spicy foods can make it much worse

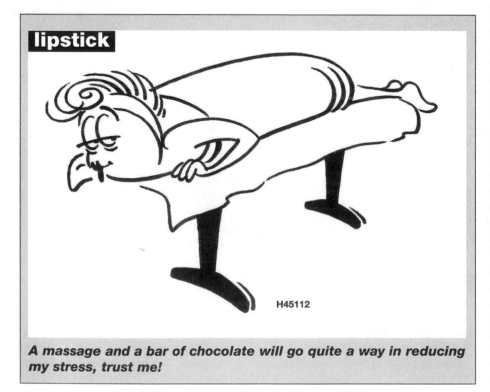

lipstick

H45112

A massage and a bar of chocolate will go quite a way in reducing my stress, trust me!

asthma (steroid inhalers do not cause ulcers) or rheumatic conditions, can cause a gastric ulcer. Even relatively small doses of anti-inflammatory drugs such as ibuprofen or aspirin can lead to an ulcer in the stomach in people who are susceptible. Duodenal ulcers are less common in women. They heal more easily than the gastric variety and usually develop just at the beginning of the duodenum.

Symptoms

2 Although symptoms vary between people there is a fairly well recognised pattern with considerable overlap between gastric and duodenal ulcers.

Gastric ulcers

• Constant pain or cramps just below the rib cage can occur which are particularly bad after eating (eating tends to settle pain in a duodenal ulcer).
• Indigestion remedies (antacids) often settle the pain but it invariably returns.
• Belching is common and embarrassing.
• Vomiting can occur and there may be black soil-like material if the ulcer is bleeding.

Duodenal ulcers

• Most people know they have developed a duodenal ulcer at around 2 am when they wake with a pain like a red hot poker just above the belly button/below the rib cage.
• Drinking milk can help but hot spicy foods can make it much worse. Eating small amounts of food often relieves the pain.

Causes

3 Ulcers may be caused by a bacterium called Helicobacter that lives in the stomach. This bacterium may also be linked to stomach cancer. There are even DIY kits available to check for this, although most cases are diagnosed by doctors. Stress, smoking and alcohol abuse may also be causative factors and can certainly make them worse.

Prevention

4 Although well treated with modern drugs it makes sense not to develop an ulcer in the first. Checking for Helicobacter is vital but avoiding smoking and excessive alcohol makes good sense. Milk and indigestion remedies (antacids) do help in the short

term but run the risk of 'rebound' where the symptoms come back with a vengeance later on. Bicarbonate of soda is highly effective but a bad idea as it turns into salt in the stomach, a major cause of high blood pressure.

Complications

5 Some things need immediate medial attention:
- Red blood or brown soil-like blood in the vomit.
- Black tar-like blood or fresh red blood in the bowel motions.
- Severe pain just below the rib cage.
- Dizziness when standing up.
- A strong thirst.

6 All of these suggest the ulcer could be bleeding or has eaten through the wall of the stomach or intestine.

Self care

7 Most peptic ulcers will respond well to treatment with modern drugs which reduce the amount of stomach acid or move it on into the intestine at a faster rate. Mild symptoms can be helped with indigestion remedies or antacids but there is no real substitute for modern medicines and clearing up any Helicobacter.

15 Piles (haemorrhoids)

1 Bums are the constant butt of jokes but piles are painful and annoying. Thankfully they are rarely serious but can make pregnancy and life after childbirth more than a tad irritating.

Symptoms

2 Pain on walking or sitting along with bleeding from the anus are the comments symptoms. The blood is often found on the toilet paper after passing a motion which can also be painful. External piles may be seen as small black grape like bodies just at the anus. Internal piles will sometimes descend through the anus only to return after passing a motion. Overzealous use of toilet paper can make things worse.

Causes

3 Some women are more likely to develop piles than others. It has nothing to do with preference of beer. More likely straining at the toilet or standing for long

periods may be factors made worse by being overweight. Constipation is probably a factor through straining at the toilet. Even lifting heavy weights has been suggested as a cause as it puts pressure on the veins near the anus. Contrary to what all of us were told at school, sitting on hot radiator pipes does not appear to cause piles.

Prevention

4 High fibre diets not only bulk up the motions they may also prevent cancer of the bowel. Similarly, taking plenty of fluids, especially fruit juices, increases the speed of the bowel. Constipation is linked to inactivity so by increasing activity it can reduce the likelihood of piles. Being overweight puts pressure on the veins near the anus in a similar way to pregnancy.

Complications

5 Pain is an obvious complication but bleeding can also occur which is more

embarrassing than dangerous. Piles can also thrombose (clot) causing even more pain and making it difficult to get them back inside the anus. Constipation can occur from not wanting to pass a motion because of the pain. This then makes passing a motion even worse. A vicious cycle.

Self care

- Ice packs really do help.
- Mini car tyres filled with cold water to sit on can restore faith in bottom range cars. (Or at last there is a use for the swimming ring that the children have grown out of using.)
- Use a bulking laxative.
- Use soft toilet paper.
- Go to the toilet on need, don't put it off.
- If passing a motion is really painful, use a lubricating, analgesic cream (obtainable from the pharmacist) an hour before going to the toilet.

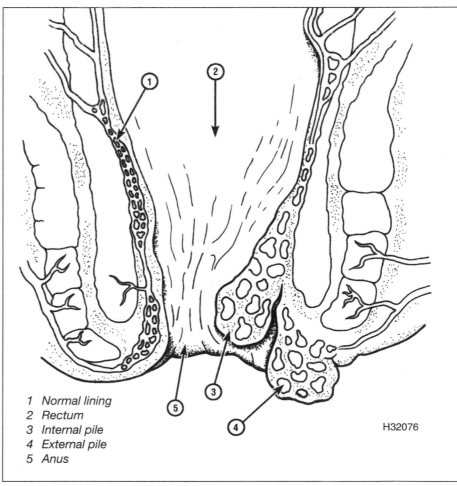

1 Normal lining
2 Rectum
3 Internal pile
4 External pile
5 Anus

H32076

15.2 Formation of piles

4

16 Raynaud's phenomenon

1 Although by no means common, many people simply put up with this condition which is a disorder affecting the small arteries supplying fingers and toes so that exposure to cold causes them to go into spasm restricting the blood supply and potentially damaging the fingers or toes.

Symptoms

2 Raynaud's disease usually affects both hands. The toes are less often affected. In cold conditions, there is tingling, burning and numbness in the affected parts and the fingers are very pale from lack of blood. (imagine coming into a warm room after being out in the bitter cold for a while).

3 As slow blood flow is resumed and the oxygen used up, the characteristic purplish colour of deoxygenated blood (cyanosis) makes the fingers or toes appear blue. When the parts are warmed and the spasm of the blood vessels passes off, the vessels open widely, allowing a flush of fresh blood to pass. In this stage, the fingers or toes become red.

Causes

4 It is not a disease in itself and occurs in any form of artery disease that causes narrowing. It can be seen for instance in people using vibrating tools.

Diagnosis

5 It is difficult to miss the characteristic physical signs (colour changes) that occur on exposure to cold. This can be replicated in the clinic to confirm the diagnosis.

Prevention

6 People suffering from Raynaud's disease must avoid cold and keep the extremities well insulated. Cigarette smoking is especially dangerous as nicotine increases the constriction of the small arteries.

Complications

7 Early on there is generally no real damage to the affected blood vessels, but in severe cases the vessel walls may eventually become thickened and the flow of blood permanently reduced. This can cause gangrene and amputation.

Treatment

8 Raynaud's phenomenon is treated by correcting the cause, if this is possible, but treatment of the symptoms may also be necessary. Various drugs to relax the smooth muscle in the walls of the arteries are useful in Raynaud's disease.

9 Cutting of the sympathetic nerves which supply the vessel wall muscles (sympathectomy) can be helpful, especially when the disease affects the lower limbs.

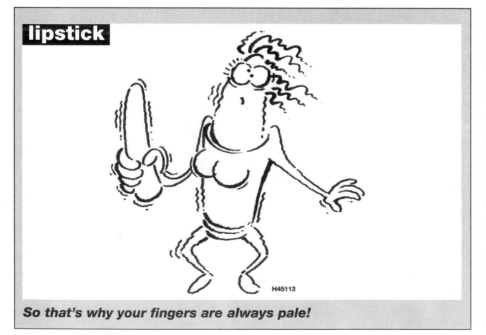

lipstick

So that's why your fingers are always pale!

17 Worms

1 Not the best topic of after-dinner conversation, worms are actually very common, particularly in children. It is not a sign of poor hygiene or bad living. Threadworms are the most common. They are itchy, embarrassing but harmless. Roundworms are larger but less common. It is also possible to be infected with worms from dogs and cats and can be more serious for younger people. Thankfully not so common, these infections can cause blindness. Tape worms were virtually extinct in the UK until the fashion for uncooked beef reintroduced the beef tape worm.

Symptoms

2 It is possible to actually see worms in the motions as tiny white/brown worms in the stool.

3 Itchy bottoms, particularly at night, are the trade mark as the female lays its eggs just at the anus at this time causing the person to scratch, pick up the eggs, and pass them on or re-infect themselves.

Causes

4 Infection with worms usually comes from contact with an infected person. They spread very quickly within a family and can remain in families for considerable periods of time without the family realising it.

Prevention

• Washing hands after going to the toilet, handling animals or working in the garden.
• Washing hands before eating.

Complications

5 Threadworms and roundworms are not serious. Worms from dogs or cats can cause blindness even in the unborn child if caught by a pregnant woman.

Self care

6 Along with the precautions stated above early treatment with worming prescriptions reduces the impact of worms but equally pets need to be wormed regularly. This is particularly important during pregnancy where contact with infected animals can be disastrous.

Chapter 5
ICE (sound and vision)

Contents

1 Ear wax

1 Ears are a marvellous invention otherwise there would be no room for the brain, and dahlias would have insects called simply called 'wigs'. Ear wax is the secretion of tiny glands called ceruminous glands in the skin of the wall of the ear's outer canal. These are modified sweat glands which produce a sticky fatty secretion protecting the eardrum by trapping dust, small objects and even insects. Normal soft wax makes its way out of the ear and is removed by washing. Hard, or dried wax tends to accumulate.

2 Some people naturally produce more than the normal amount of wax. Those who do so sometimes suffer deafness from total blockage of the ear canal. Harsh syringing can makes things worse as anything that irritates the ear canal will produce more wax than before, so removal of wax by syringing can give

great relief but this should be done by an expert aware of the risks. It is also better to avoid syringing, in case infected material should be carried into the middle ear through an unseen perforation in the ear drum.

Symptoms

3 Deafness is not caused by wax until the ear canal is completely obstructed, but this may occur suddenly if water gets into the ears lodging between the wax and the ear drum. Ear wax absorbs water and swells up.

Causes and prevention

4 The rate of secretion of wax is affected by irritation to the skin, and constant poking of the ears with paperclips, cotton buds, toothpicks or other objects will tend to produce more wax.

5 If hard wax is a problem, the application of a little olive oil (not multigrade) will help to soften it. Proprietary wax softening products are also available from the pharmacist.

2 Hearing loss

1 Unfortunately there is more than one way to suffer a hearing loss. The commonest way is exposure to continuous loud noise. 'Disco Deafness' is self explanatory but the noise doesn't need to be so loud. Even personal stereo headphones will cause damage to the hearing if used at too high a volume, and will probably be known as 'Mobile Middle Ear' with the present explosion in mobile phones and personal stereos. Infection is another factor although infection of the middle ear and so called 'glue' ear are no longer thought to be a major cause of permanent hearing loss. Ear wax is the commonest cause of temporary deafness, made worse by attempts to remove it with a cotton bud. This has about the same degree of success as trying to take a cannon ball out of a cannon with a ramrod.

5

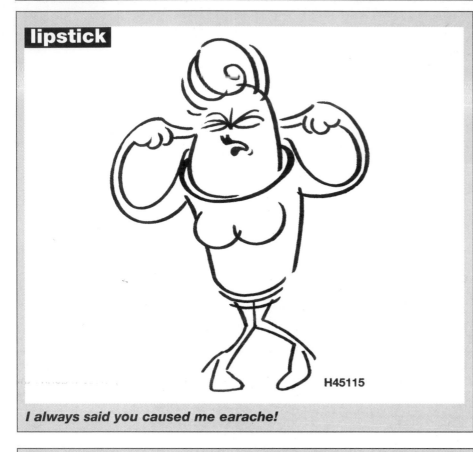

I always said you caused me earache!

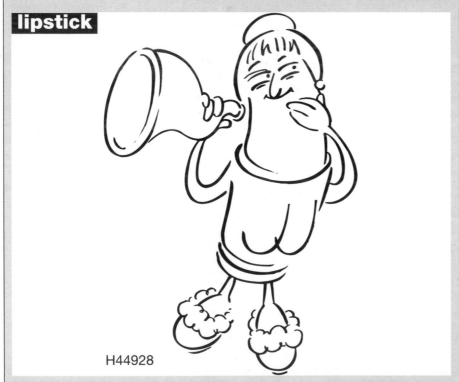

Loss of hearing can cause accidents and potentially dangerous misunderstandings over instructions

Symptoms

2 Hearing is taken for granted and a gradual hearing loss is usually missed or ignored until there is difficulty hearing speech. By this time the damage has invariably been done, particularly if it was caused by prolonged and repeated exposure to loud noise. There may also be a ringing or hissing noise (tinnitus) much worse when in a quiet room or at night. Less often there may also be dizziness (vertigo) although this tends to occur while the damage is taking place.

Causes

3 Prolonged exposure to loud noise is a common cause, particularly in industry and farming. Increasingly women are working in environments previously the sole domain of men. Sadly they are often suffering from the effects of such harsh surroundings.

4 Some viral infections may cause deafness and tinnitus. There are basically two types of deafness.

• Conductive deafness involves the poor conduction of sound from the ear drum, along the middle ear bones (ossicles) and on to the sensory structure which converts the sound vibrations into nerve impulses for the brain to understand (cochlea). Diseases which attack the ear drum or middle ear bones reduce their ability to conduct sound.

• Perceptive deafness involves the cochlea or auditory nerve and this permanent damage is commonly caused by loud noise exposure.

Prevention

5 While it might not be possible to prevent most diseases of the ear, preventing hearing loss through wearing ear protectors and using sound baffles is relatively easy. Using headsets which have a maximum safe volume is also advisable as there is otherwise a temptation to steadily increase the volume.

Complications

6 Loss of hearing can cause accidents and potentially dangerous misunderstandings over instructions. It can be a terrible social barrier for some people. Some forms of deafness are accompanied by tinnitus which can be very distressing. Consult your GP in the first instance, who will probably refer you to a specialist.

Self care

7 The smallest thing you should ever put in the ear is the elbow. Never attempt to physically remove wax. Instead use wax softeners obtainable from the pharmacist, or olive oil. Avoid syringing as much as possible; it tends to stimulate the production of more wax and can pass infection into the middle ear if there is an ear drum perforation.

3 Middle ear infection (acute otitis media)

1 There few more irritating pains than those which can accompany infections of the middle ear. Worse still they are common although tending to decrease with age. Historically these were considered potentially life threatening as mastoiditis (a serious bone infection of the skull) was often linked. For whatever reason mastoiditis is now very rare and middle ear infections are not considered quite so serious as before. Even so, they are very painful and can cause a temporary loss of hearing. A recent cold or throat infection may have happened before the pain in the ear started.

Symptoms

2 Most people complain of a dullness in their hearing as if there was cotton wool blocking their ear. There is also a severe throbbing pain made worse sometimes by sneezing, coughing or blowing their nose. If there is pus behind the ear drum it may leak through a small hole, not unlike a boil on the skin. Once the pus escapes the pain rapidly declines. It is difficult not to notice this happening as the pus usually flows out very quickly and has a strong smell. The ear drum repairs itself within a short space of time once all the pus has drained and there is very rarely any loss of hearing as a result.

Causes

3 Infections of the tube which connects the ear to the back of the throat – the Eustachian tube – may help cause middle ear infections. This tends to happen during cold or flu epidemics. Its job is to keep the pressures equal on both sides of the ear drum, pressure builds up in the middle ear which is the main cause of pain.

Prevention

4 Some doctors feel that mentholated pastilles sucked during a cold may prevent the Eustachian tube from blocking but there is no hard evidence to support this. Smoking may increase the risk as it can inflame the narrow tube.

Complications

5 It was once thought that middle ear infections caused permanent loss of hearing. This is no longer considered completely true. Repeated infections with persistent rupture through the ear drum can cause scarring which stiffens the thin ear drum, reducing its sensitivity to sound.

Self care

6 Pain relief is the main treatment as antibiotics take a long time to take effect and may not be of any real value. Paracetamol will reduce the pain and hard swallowing should be encouraged rather than blowing against a pinched nose to help unblock the Eustachian tube.

4 Tinnitus

1 Although this basically means noise in the ear, it has many different forms and affects different people very differently. It is also common but for many people they only begin to notice it in later life. The sounds people hear also varies, about 25 per cent of people with tinnitus experience musical noises while the rest describe it as hissing, buzzing or ringing.

2 Nearly everyone has experienced short periods of singing in the ears. This may be spontaneous or due to a loud noise, a cold or a blow on the head. In established tinnitus, the sound is continuous, but sufferers are not always aware of it, so that it appears to be intermittent. It is often worst in bed at night, probably because there is then less background noise. It is, to a variable extent, masked by external background noises that are usually present during the day.

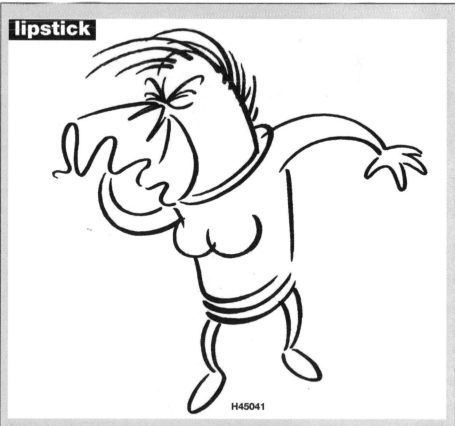

lipstick

H45041

Mother always told me not to blow hard when I had a cold. See, Mother does know best!

5

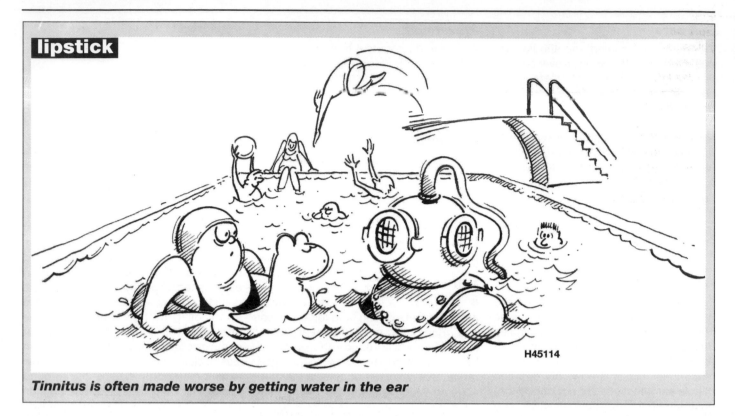

lipstick

Tinnitus is often made worse by getting water in the ear

Causes

3 Tinnitus is almost always associated with some degree of deafness and is related to damage to the hair cells of the cochlea of the inner ear. These delicate hair cells are the means by which acoustic vibrations are converted into nerve impulses for passage to the brain.

4 Tinnitus can be caused by any of the factors known to cause deafness, such as:

• Nearby explosions (even balloons bursting can cause temporary tinnitus).
• A blow on the ear.
• Prolonged loud noise (this includes discos and raves).
• Fracture of the base of the skull (can happen from simply jumping off a high wall or parachuting).
• Tumour in the nerve from the ear to the brain (acoustic neuroma).
• Some antibiotics.
• Diuretic drugs.
• Quinine (don't forget tonic water which contains quite a bit of quinine to give the sharp taste).
• Various ear disorders, such as Menière's disease, otosclerosis, labyrinthitis and presbyacusis.

5 Nearby loud noises (acoustic trauma) are among the most important causes of tinnitus and deafness. The risks of noise-induced damage to hearing should be more widely known. After exposure to noise loud enough to cause temporary deafness, most of the hearing loss is restored, usually in a matter of hours; but some permanent loss occurs.

6 This damage is the result of structural injury to the delicate hair cells. The degree of permanent damage depends on the noise intensity and on the length of exposure.

7 The causes of temporary tinnitus include:

• Ear wax irritating the eardrum (often made worse by getting water in the ear as well).
• Middle ear infection (otitis media).
• Glue ear (serous otitis media but seen mainly in children).
• Impacted wisdom teeth (infections underneath the molar teeth can spread through the bone and inflame the inner ear).

8 Thankfully all of these are treatable and none is likely to lead to permanent tinnitus.

Treatment

9 Certain drugs, such as local anaesthetics and others which interfere with nerve conduction, have been found to have an effect on tinnitus. Distraction is the best strategy. Some people have found it helpful to listen to low-level music on personal headphones. Others have invested in 'white noise' generators (tinnitus maskers). These produce a rival sound on which to concentrate.

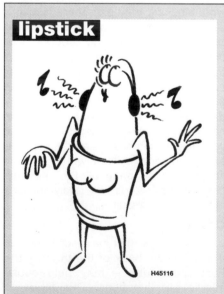

lipstick

My doctor says I need a personal stereo. Yes, really – I'm not a fashion victim, it's medically prescribed!

5 Conjunctivitis

1 The eye is an amazingly tough organ but it is vulnerable to inflammation of the transparent covering over the eye, the conjunctiva. Infection, foreign bodies, constant rubbing or chemical irritation are all causes. People with allergies to plants or certain chemicals may inadvertently cause conjunctivitis by rubbing their eyes after handling the substances. In most cases the Inflammation will subside on its own.

Symptoms

2 With inflammation the blood vessels in the conjunctiva enlarge and the eye may appear 'bloodshot'. If there is infection, pus may collect during the night under the eyelid and can matt the two eye lids together. Bacterial infections, reactions to chemicals or allergies often affect both eyes whereas viral infections tend only to affect one eye, at least initially. Pus is much less of a feature with allergic or chemical reactions. Instead there can be a quite dramatic swelling of the conjunctiva producing a boggy jelly like effect around the centre of the eye which remains unaffected. It will settle on its own although it can be treated with anti-inflammatory eye drops.

Causes

3 Some infections are very contagious and bacteria from another infected person, often a member of the family or a school child, can be passed on through sharing towels or even physical contact. Viral infections can also arise spontaneously. Grass and pollen will irritate the eye, especially if where there is already hay fever allergy. Wood resin, household chemicals, petrol, and many other common substance will also cause conjunctivitis. A common cause is hot pepper sauces which can cause pain as well as inflammation.

Prevention

4 Using separate towels and face clothes while a relation is infected makes good sense. Wear goggles when handling chemicals. Antihistamines really do make a difference during high pollen counts for hay fever sufferer.

Complications

5 Corneal grafting. Viral infections are more serious if they are on the transparent centre of the eye, not the conjunctiva. This can be seen in herpetic infections on the face which reach as far as the tip of the nose. This is a good indication that the eye has become involved as well.

Self care

6 Antibiotic drops prescribed by a doctor will clear bacterial infections but it can take up to a week for the infection to clear and things are made much better by gently cleaning the crusted pus away from the eyelids with cotton wool and warm water. Do not use the same cloth on the other eye and use only once for each wipe. Viral infections need prompt and frequent treatment with anti-viral drops and should be seen by a consultant ophthalmologist. Antihistamine drops can make a dramatic difference for allergic conjunctivitis and are available from the pharmacist without a prescription.

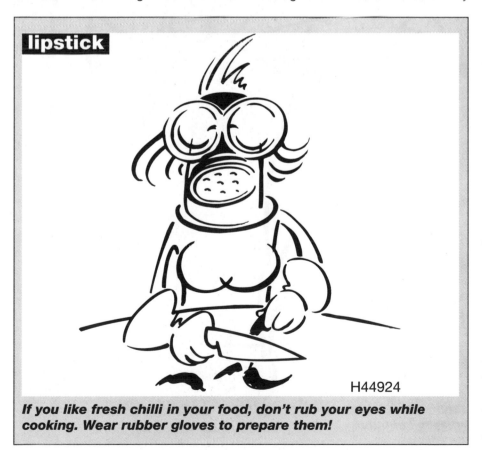

lipstick

H44924

If you like fresh chilli in your food, don't rub your eyes while cooking. Wear rubber gloves to prepare them!

6 Glaucoma

1 The eyeball is a contradiction. The outer coat of the eyeball is tough but soft. Unless the pressure of the fluid within it were maintained, it would gently collapse like a balloon with a slow puncture. All round the back of the root of the iris of the eye there are cells that continuously produce a fluid of almost pure water called aqueous humour which keeps the eyeball in a firm shape. Should the pressure of aqueous humour increase too high the small blood vessels within the eye would be compressed, cutting off vital oxygen to the retina and damaging normal vision.

2 Exit ports around the iris filter the excess fluid out of the eyeball so that between the rate of production of the water and the rate of exit, the pressure in the eyeball is normally kept at a safe level.

3 Glaucoma is a group of eye diseases in which the pressure of the fluid within the eyeball is too high. This can happen

5

in two ways. Either the tiny openings in the outlet filter can get partially blocked, or the iris can move forward to obstruct access to the filter. These two possibilities are the causes of the two main kinds of glaucoma.

4 Chronic simple glaucoma, the commonest form, is a major cause of blindness. If detected early, the pressures can be controlled and the damage stopped. Unfortunately, the condition is very gradual and completely painless, and the fibres first affected are those coming from the outer part of the retina. Loss of peripheral parts of the visual field is very difficult to notice. This is the type carried in families.

5 About one person in 100 has glaucoma at the age of 40, but the incidence rises steeply with increasing age. By the age of 70, about one person in ten has significantly raised eye pressures. Chronic simple glaucoma runs in families and is more likely to occur in relatives of people with the disease. Only in the late stages will there be obvious symptoms. As peripheral vision is the first to be damaged and central vision usually the last to go, one eye may be completely blinded before it is appreciated that anything is wrong.

6 However, in other, less common, forms of glaucoma, the pressure rise is caused in different ways. The effects may be more obvious. In the most severe form the symptoms may be dramatic, with great pain and sudden loss of all vision. This is the case in acute congestive glaucoma or in glaucoma caused by eye disease where blockages occur because of inflammation.

Symptoms

7 Unfortunately, chronic simple glaucoma produces almost no symptoms until it is at an advanced stage at which much of the outer (peripheral) field of vision has been lost. Surprisingly, very few people notice the loss of peripheral vision. Driving is hazardous and they may notice that they are constantly bumping into others on busy pavements, but fail to realize why.

8 A less severe and less common form, called sub-acute glaucoma, causes symptoms that should be more easily recognized. These usually occur at night when the pupils are wide. There is a dull aching pain in the eye, some fogginess of vision, and, characteristically, concentric, rainbow-coloured rings are seen around lights. The condition can easily be prevented by the use of eye drops and is curable by a simple operation or outpatient laser procedure.

9 The symptoms of the least common but most dangerous form, acute glaucoma, are so severe there is little room for doubt that something is not right. The affected eye is acutely painful, red, hard and tender to the touch. The pupil is often enlarged even in dim light and the normally transparent cornea steamy and partly opaque. The vision is grossly diminished. Urgent treatment is needed to reduce the pressure, so no time must be wasted. Ring 999/112 or go directly to A&E.

Causes

10 The fibres concerned with vision at the extreme outer limits of fields of vision are damaged, possibly destroyed permanently but it is hard to notice that peripheral vision has been lost. This is because the brain concentrates on a narrow area around the point observed. Many people can lose extensive peripheral vision without being aware of it.

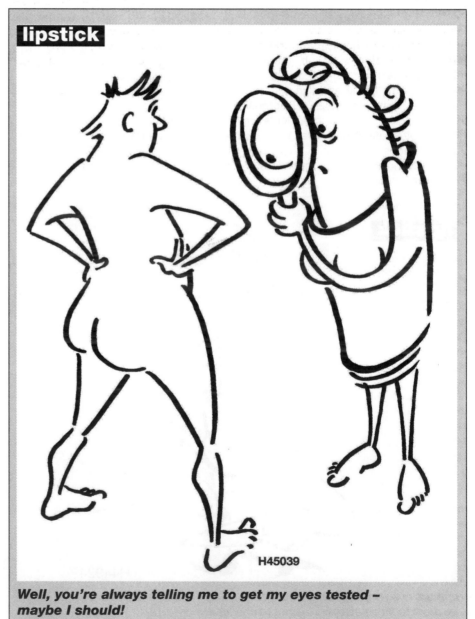

lipstick

H45039

Well, you're always telling me to get my eyes tested – maybe I should!

Diagnosis

11 The best test is to measure the internal pressure by a simple technique known as tonometry. The measuring device (tonometer) is mounted on a slit-lamp – a low-power microscope with a brilliant light source used to examine the eye. After local anaesthetic drops the soft cup of the tonometer is pressed against the eye. A direct reading of the internal eye pressure can be made from the force needed to gently dent the eyeball's outer surface. It is neither uncomfortable or painful.

Complications

12 The complication of undetected, untreated glaucoma is blindness and is one of the principal reasons for people needing to register as blind. Chronic simple glaucoma is the most likely to remain undetected before a late stage.

Treatment

13 Glaucoma must first be detected, then treated. In most cases the pressures can be kept under control by regular daily use of eye drops, usually beta blockers, that reduce the rate of production of aqueous humour within the eye. If eye drops fail, some form of surgery will be necessary.

14 Laser trabeculoplasty is a treatment for glaucoma, using a laser to burn several tiny holes in the outflow filter of the eye, the trabecular meshwork. This causes scars that, on contraction, widen the channels of the meshwork and make it easier for the aqueous humour to flow out and reduce the pressure in the eye.

15 Trabeculectomy is an operation on the sclera to provide an alternative route for fluid drainage out of the eye, so as to reduce the pressure and prevent further damage. The membrane covering the sclera, the conjunctiva, is opened behind the upper eyelid. A tiny square flap of half-thickness sclera is raised and a permanent opening is made through the inner half-thickness.

16 The outer flap is now returned to its original position and its free corners secured each with a single tiny stitch. The conjunctiva is securely closed. Aqueous humour is now able to escape from the eye through the edges of the outer flap and pass under the conjunctiva from which location it is absorbed into the blood.

17 The simple message is to check regularly.

Chapter 6
Family runabout

Contents

1 Cancer of the cervix

See Chapter 7.

2 Pre-menstrual problems (PMS)

1 PMS is one of the most baffling phenomena for men. It is well known that testosterone drives young men to inexplicable behaviour but it tends to be a temporary phase. PMS on the other hand has a cycle which is often lost on men but will be condemned for explaining any similar behaviour in women. Still, myths abound and jokes, often thinly disguised sexism, litter the internet. Women were once barred from driving and riding horses during the pre-menstrual period. It has even been used successfully as a defence in court. In truth, not all women suffer from pre-menstrual syndrome but for those that do, and up to 40% of women still menstruating will, it can be a distressing time of the month. The severity of the syndrome varies between women and even from month to month. It is also known as pre-menstrual tension (PMT).

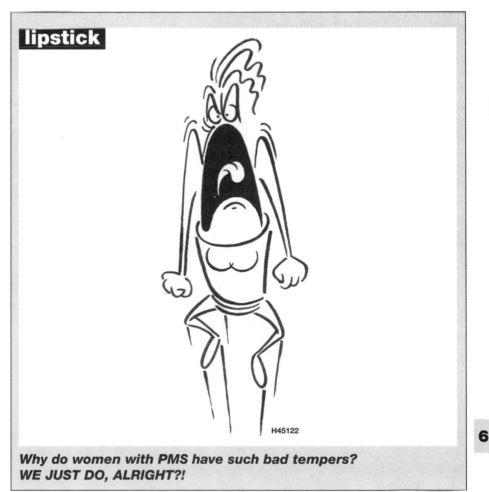

lipstick

Why do women with PMS have such bad tempers? WE JUST DO, ALRIGHT?!

Symptoms

- Depression without apparent cause.
- Irritability and anxiety.
- Tiredness.
- Tender breasts.
- Headache.
- Water retention (thick ankles, especially at night, increased waist size).
- Paranoia (feelings of hostility and anger).
- Desire for certain foods.

Causes

2 It is normal and hormone changes are probably a factor. Women on the oral contraceptive pill, for instance, often report a reduction in symptoms. What value it has in evolution is unclear, discouraging men from sexual contact during menses may have an advantage in preventing infection and many cultures expressly forbid it, but good evidence is thin on the ground. The level of steroid hormones affects water retention and many women report an increase in weight along with 'bloating'. There is no standard level of PMS as it varies considerably in severity between women.

Self care

- Avoiding caffeine-containing drinks can help but it is worth remembering that tea can contain as much as coffee. Conversely, some women find tea a boon.
- Eating lightly, more often, seems to reduce the severity of the symptoms for some women.
- A reduced salt intake can certainly help reduce water retention.
- Remaining or even increasing the level of activity may also help.

3 PMS is often the great excuse and explanation for more serious states of mind. It can, for instance be confused with depression. Feelings of self harm need the attention of a doctor.

3 Period pain (dysmenorrhoea)

1 Although many women suffer from period pain its severity can vary enormously between women from very mild to severe. The pain may also vary between monthly cycles. The good news is that generally speaking, it gets better with age and after pregnancy.

Symptoms

- Cramping abdominal pains.
- Backache.
- General fatigue.
- Nausea & vomiting.
- Diarrhoea.
- Headaches.
- Pre-menstrual bloating (water retention).

Causes

2 The causes of severe period pain can be numerous but there are basically two types of period pain:

Primary

- Mainly seen in girls/women who have just begun to have periods (menstruate). The pain and discomfort may disappear or become less severe after a woman leaves teenagehood or gives birth. Hormones such as prostaglandins are closely involved with the cramping sensation and can cause a spasm of the uterus.

Secondary

- This is period pain that is due to other disorders of the reproductive system, such as fibroids, endometriosis, ovarian cysts and, rarely, cancer. Intrauterine devices (IUD), can also increase period pain, especially in women who have never been pregnant.

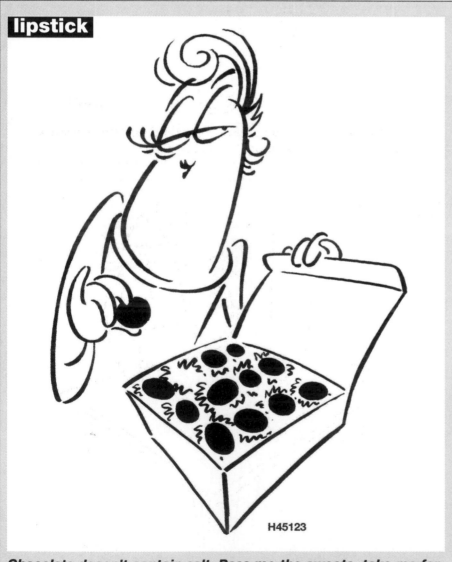

lipstick

H45123

Chocolate doesn't contain salt. Pass me the sweets, take me for a walk and make like you're on eggshells, boy!

• Oral contraceptives reduce painful periods in 70 to 80% of women and there are preparations which do not act as a contraceptive but the hormones they contain help reduce period pain, especially in endometriosis (see *Endometriosis*). If this type of pill is used some other form of contraception (eg, condoms) must also be used.

Prevention

3 Recognising when the pains are about to start (see PMS) can give you chance to start medication early thus reducing the severity of the pain.

Complications

4 Obviously uncomplicated period pain is a normal part of the female reproductive cycle but that doesn't mean women should suffer. Any underlying condition which is making things worse needs medical attention.

Self care

5 Anti-inflammatory drugs such as aspirin or ibuprofen relieve pain and inhibit the release of prostaglandins. Although paracetamol will help ease the pain it will not inhibit the release of prostaglandins and is generally not as effective for this reason.

• Hot drinks such as warm milk or lemon and honey seem to help some women.

• Tucking the legs in while lying down helps ease the cramps.

• Hot-water bottles have long been used to ease pain especial during periods.

• Long restful warm baths ease the stress as well as the pain.

• As with muscular pain generally, gentle massage of the lower abdomen can increase blood flow and ease the pain. Similarly for exercise which also acts as a distraction.

• Some women find an orgasm can help with period pain – with him or on their own.

Ring your GP/NHS Direct if there is:

• Period pain unlike any other time and it is getting worse.

• Any abnormal vaginal discharge along with the pain.

• Pain starting sooner and taking longer to depart.

• Pain is occurring in between periods as well.

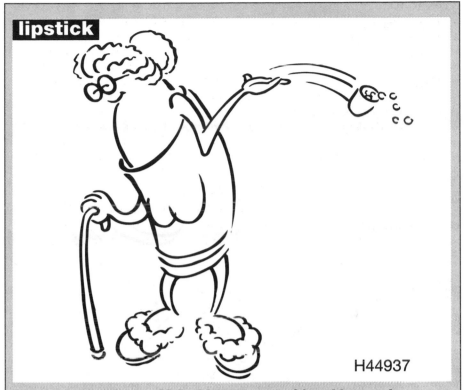

lipstick

H44937

That's the good news?? So I have to get old and have a house full of sprogs to stop the pain? Nooooooo!

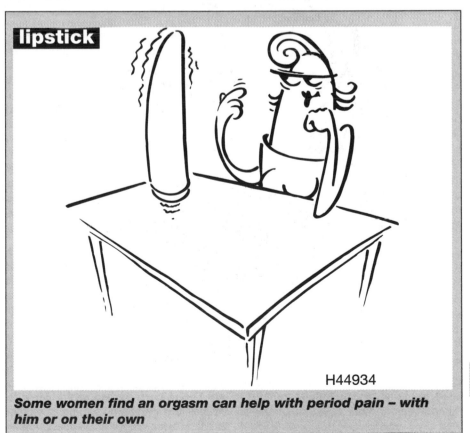

lipstick

H44934

Some women find an orgasm can help with period pain – with him or on their own

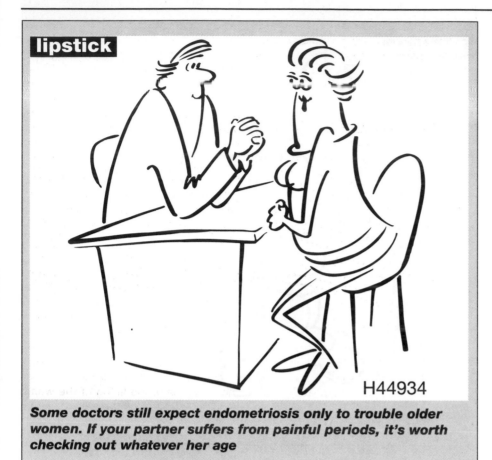

lipstick

H44934

Some doctors still expect endometriosis only to trouble older women. If your partner suffers from painful periods, it's worth checking out whatever her age

4 Endometriosis

1 For centuries women have reported bleeding during their periods from places like the nose. Difficult to explain until the structure of the womb was worked out. The lining of the womb (uterus) is called the endometrium. Each month this layer of cells grows in size then is shed with the period. These cells should normally only be found lining the womb but in some cases they migrate to different parts of the body, usually the inside of the abdomen. They still respond to the hormonal changes which take place every month and will bleed despite being in the wrong place. This produces cysts around the area. More rarely they lodge in other parts of the body.

Symptoms

2 Most women will not be aware of endometriosis as thankfully most of these cells will not cause any major problems but they can cause severe abdominal or back pain which gradually gets worse as each period approaches. There may be heavy periods with large amounts of blood loss so anaemia can be a problem. Sexual intercourse can also be painful especially near the time of a period.

Causes

3 The endometrial cells will only cause these problems before menopause as they shrivel away without the promoting influence of female hormones so it is more common between the ages of 30 and 40 years.
4 Some doctors still expect endometriosis only to trouble older women. If your partner suffers from painful periods, it's worth checking out whatever her age.

Prevention

5 Although the reason remains obscure, having children appears to reduce the risk from endometriosis.

Complications

6 The commonest complication is simply pain but reduced fertility, ectopic pregnancy and depression may result from severe endometriosis.

Treatment

7 Herbal treatments are advocated by some but hormones, given by mouth, injection, nasal spray or skin patch may help reduce the activity of the endometrial cells until menopause. In severe cases surgery using laser or electrocautery can reduce the symptoms of endometriosis by removing the bulk of the cells.

5 Fibroids

1 Myths abound around the womb, particularly fibroids. They are not a result of promiscuity, alcohol abuse or pregnancies that did not go through to completion. These growths are benign tumours of the womb and are not malignant. They form within the wall of the uterus (womb), on the outside or inside the womb itself. Their size varies as does the speed at which they grow which can be from pea sized to golf ball. Although most common in women around 45 years old, around 20% of women aged 30 years or over will have fibroids.

Symptoms

2 Most women are completely unaware of fibroids, especially if the fibroids are very small. For some women however there can be prolonged, heavy and painful periods. In rare cases it can be felt as a hard lump in the lower abdomen and if it presses on the bladder it may cause pain on passing water or during sexual intercourse.

Causes

3 The cause of fibroids is not known. There may be a genetic factor but it seems in the main that they are common in all women irrespective of social class or ethnicity.

Prevention

4 There is no known way to prevent fibroids; it used to be thought that early pregnancy reduced the risk.

Complications

5 Fibroids were often removed unnecessarily but actually they only

rarely cause pain from a lack of blood supply requiring an operation to remove them. If fibroids grow large enough they can prevent conception and may even cause miscarriage. The good news is that fibroids tend to decrease in size with age over 45 years so are probably sensitive to hormone levels.

6 Contraception

1 There are numerous methods of contraception, most of which, it has to be said, depend more on the woman than the man. Not only is there a difference in the way the methods work and are used, but there is a significant difference in the protection each method provides.

The male condom

2 Society is increasingly accepting the condom as one of the normal requirements of modern life. This has led to their wider availability and condoms can now readily be obtained – in supermarkets, from garages, by mail order, through slot machines, as well as in pharmacies. They are free from all family planning clinics and genito-urinary medicine clinics. Colours, flavours and new materials, like plastic, make interesting options. Condoms now come in different shapes and sizes, and it is often necessary to try a few different types before the right one is found. If used correctly condoms are 98% effective at preventing pregnancy and they have the added advantage of providing good protection against many sexually transmitted infections. Hermetically sealed, the modern condom will remain usable for a long time (look for the expiry date); good quality condoms will also have the CE mark and the kitemark. Once the seal is broken they should be used quite soon as the rubber will perish on exposure to the air and the lubricant will dry, making it difficult to put on.

3 Using a condom correctly is essential for it to be effective. It should be put on before any contact between the penis and the vagina or genital area, and rolled on the correct way round. Air should be excluded from the end of the condom as it can cause it to burst or slip off. Sharp

finger nails, rings and teeth are a hazard. Only the soft finger pulps should be used to unroll the condom on to the penis. If extra lubrication is needed then only a water based one should be used with rubber condoms. There is a need to withdraw and remove the condom while the penis is still erect to avoid semen leaking out as the penis shrinks in size.

4 Perhaps the single biggest stated reason for not using condoms is the widely held belief that they inhibit spontaneous sex. Foreplay is an important part of enjoyable sexual activity and partners can involve the condom in this. Fears that they reduce the sensitivity of sexual experience have not been supported by research. Most of the problem is with the psychological inhibition some men have over their use but without doubt lots of foreplay does help.

The female condom

5 The condom for women is relatively new, but regular users report favourably and many men prefer them to the male condom. Made of plastic it is larger in diameter than the male condom and has a flexible ring at each end. The smaller ring fits inside the vagina while the outer, larger, ring remains on the outside of the vagina. After ejaculation this outer ring should be twisted to prevent escape of the sperm and the condom gently withdrawn. Female condoms are 95% effective, and also have the advantage of providing protection against many sexually transmitted infections.

Oral contraception (the Pill)

6 The combined pill contains two hormones which inhibit the release of the hormones which stimulate the final development and release of ova (eggs) from the ovary. This partly mimics a pregnancy, which explains why some women suffer the milder symptoms of being pregnant when using this pill.

7 The combined pill is convenient, over 99% effective when taken correctly, and has many advantages (including protection against cancer of the womb and the ovary). Like all drugs, there are health risks associated with its use. A very small number of women will develop a blood clot which can be life-threatening. Women who take the pill are also more at risk of being diagnosed with

breast cancer or cervical cancer. However, for the vast majority of women the advantages of taking the pill greatly outweigh the risks.

8 The progestogen-only pill contains only one hormone and stops sperm from getting anywhere near the egg by maintaining the natural plug of mucus in the neck of the womb. It also makes the lining of the womb thinner. It is highly effective (99%) and it is particularly useful for women who cannot use the combined pill, and those who are breast feeding. It has, however, to be taken regularly at the same time each day, and can have the disadvantage of causing irregular bleeding.

Intrauterine contraceptive device (IUD)

9 These small plastic and copper devices are inserted into the womb by GPs, or by doctors or nurses at family planning clinics. They prevent pregnancy by stopping the sperm and egg meeting; they also make the lining of the womb unsuitable for implantation should fertilisation occur. They are over 99% effective, can be left in place for up to eight years, and can be used by women both before and after having children. They are not suitable for women who are at risk of getting a sexually transmitted infection, and can make periods longer and heavier. To minimise the risk of infection, tests are done before the IUD is put in. The IUD is removed very easily by a doctor or nurse and has no effect upon sensation during intercourse.

Intrauterine contraceptive system (IUS)

10 These small plastic T-shaped devices contain the hormone progestogen. They are inserted into the womb by GPs, or by doctors or nurses at family planning clinics. They prevent pregnancy in the same way as the progestogen-only pill. They are over 99% effective, can be left in place for up to five years, and can be used by women both before and after having children. Initial side-effects can include irregular bleeding, but periods then tend to become lighter and shorter, or stop altogether; period pain is also reduced. Like the IUD, the IUS is removed very easily by a doctor or nurse and has no effect upon sensation during intercourse.

6

CONTRACEPTIVE METHODS WITH POSSIBILITY OF USER FAILURE
The methods in this table must be used correctly to achieve the effectiveness stated.

	Combined pill	Progestogen-only pill	Male condom	Female condom	Diaphragm or cap	Natural family planning (NFP)
How it works	Contains two hormones, oestrogen and progestogen, which stop ovulation.	Contains the hormone progestogen, which thickens the cervical mucus, and stops sperm getting near the egg.	Barrier method. The condom covers the penis and stops sperm entering the vagina.	Barrier method. The condom lines the vagina and stops sperm entering.	Barrier method. A rubber or silicone cap covers the cervix to keep sperm out of the womb. Used with spermicidal cream or jelly.	Fertile and infertile times in the menstrual cycle are identified.
Pros	Can reduce PMS, period pain and bleeding. Protects against cancer of the womb and ovary.	Can be used when breast-feeding. More suitable for older smokers than the combined pill.	Wide choice and easy availability. Provides some protection against sexually transmitted infections. Under male control.	Can be put in before sex. Provides some protection against sexually transmitted infections.	Can be put in before sex. Provides some protection against sexually transmitted infections.	Freedom from side-effects. Awareness of fertile times can be used for planning pregnancies as well as avoiding them.
Cons	Increased risk of breast and cervical cancer. Increased risk of thrombosis (blood clots).	May produce irregular periods with bleeding in between. May be less effective in women weighing over 70 kg (11 stone).	Need to stop to put it on. Can split or come off if not used correctly. Need to withdraw while still erect.	If not inserted in advance, need to stop to put it in. Need to make sure that the penis enters correctly.	If not inserted in advance, need to stop to put it in. Can provoke cystitis in some users.	Method must be taught by a qualified teacher. Users must abstain from sex, or use a barrier method, during the fertile period.
Remarks	Smokers over 35 should not use it (risk of thrombosis).	Must be taken at exactly the same time each day (to within 3 hours).	Do not re-use. Must be put on before genital contact occurs. Do not use oil-based lubricants on latex condoms.	Do not re-use. Must be put in before genital contact occurs. Expensive to buy, but can be obtained free at some family planning clinics.	Must be correctly fitted, and fit must be checked every 12 months. Must be put in before genital contact occurs.	There are various different methods of indicating fertility. Effectiveness is highest when using several indicators.
Effectiveness*	Over 99%	99%	98%	95%	92% to 96%	Up to 98%

* Effectiveness is expressed as the percentage of women who will not get pregnant with each year of correct use of a particular contraceptive method. So if the effectiveness is 99%, 1 woman in 100 will get pregnant in a year. Using no contraception at all, 80 to 90 women out of 100 will get pregnant in a year.

CONTRACEPTIVE METHODS WITH NO POSSIBILITY OF USER FAILURE

The effectiveness of the methods in this table does not depend on the user.

	Contraceptive injection	Implant	Intrauterine system (IUS)	Intrauterine device (IUD)	Female sterilisation	Male sterilisation (vasectomy)
How it works	The hormone progestogen is slowly released, stopping ovulation and thickening the cervical mucus.	An implant is placed under the skin. It releases the hormone progestogen, stopping ovulation and thickening the cervical mucus.	A small plastic device is inserted into the womb. It releases the hormone progestogen, thickening the cervical mucus.	A small plastic and copper device is inserted into the womb. It stops sperm meeting an egg, or fertilised eggs implanting.	The fallopian tubes are cut, sealed or otherwise blocked. The egg cannot meet the sperm.	The tubes carrying the sperm from each testis are cut or blocked. There are no sperm in the semen.
Pros	Single injection lasts for 8 or 12 weeks. Protects against cancer of the womb and ovary.	Single implant works for 3 years. Quickly reversed at any time.	Single insertion lasts for 5 years. Quickly reversed at any time. Periods are normally lighter and less painful.	Single insertion lasts for up to 10 years (depending on model). Effective immediately.	Permanent. No known long-term side-effects.	Permanent. No known long-term side-effects. Minor operation under local anaesthetic.
Cons	Fertility may take a year to return after stopping the injections. Periods may become irregular or stop. Other side-effects, including weight gain, in some users.	Periods may become irregular or stop. Other side-effects, including weight gain, in some users.	Irregular light bleeding for the first 3 months is common; sometimes this lasts longer. Other side-effects in some users.	Periods may become, heavier, longer and more painful. Not suitable for women at risk of catching a sexually transmitted infection.	Invasive surgical procedure under general anaesthetic. Small possibility (1 in 200) of tubes rejoining and restoring fertility.	Expect some swelling and discomfort after the operation. Very small possibility (1 in 2000) of tubes rejoining.
Remarks	Effects cannot be stopped until the injection runs out.	Usually inserted and removed using a local anaesthetic.	Useful for women with very heavy or painful periods.	IUD insertion can also be used as emergency contraception.	Should be assumed to be irreversible. Other contraception must be used until the first period after sterilisation.	Should be assumed to be irreversible. Other contraception must be used until there have been two consecutive negative sperm tests.
Effectiveness*	Over 99%	Over 99%	Over 99%	98% or better	99.5%	99.95%

* Effectiveness is expressed as the percentage of women who will not get pregnant with each year of correct use of a particular contraceptive method. So if the effectiveness is 99%, 1 woman in 100 will get pregnant in a year. Using no contraception at all, 80 to 90 women out of 100 will get pregnant in a year.

Hormone implant (for women)

11 One small rod containing progestogen is inserted under the skin in the arm, usually using a local anaesthetic. It works like the progestogen-only pill and lasts for three years. The main disadvantage is that it can cause irregular bleeding for several months. It is over 99% effective and is easily removed in a minute or two.

Hormone injection (for women)

12 The hormone progestogen is given as an injection every 8 or 12 weeks, depending on the type used. It is over 99% effective and works by stopping the ovaries producing eggs. It shares many of the advantages of the combined pill, but can cause irregular bleeding and weight gain. Once the injections stop it can take a year or more for periods to return.

The male Pill

13 The day when a male pill will be available slowly gets nearer. There have been successful human trials in the UK, and in the next decade we should see a male hormonal method of contraception. At the moment it is unclear whether this will be in the form of a pill, an implant or an injection.

Female sterilisation

14 This is a permanent method of contraception in which the fallopian tubes are either cut, sealed or blocked so that eggs cannot pass down them to the uterus (womb). It has a failure rate of 1 in 200, making it 99.5% effective – as good as other long-term reversible methods. Should it fail, it carries a greater risk of the egg implanting in the fallopian tube (ectopic pregnancy). As a general anaesthetic is required and the operation is more invasive it is a more complicated and risky procedure than vasectomy. It is possible to reverse the operation but with limited success, and with an increased risk of ectopic pregnancy.

Emergency contraception

15 'Emergency' contraception is a safe and effective way of preventing pregnancy. It involves either taking tablets containing progestogen (which are used within 72 hours of sex but are more effective the sooner they are taken) or inserting an IUD. Emergency methods can be used when no contraception was used or when regular contraception has failed.

Emergency pills are safe to take and have no lasting effects on future fertility. Emergency contraception is available free from GPs, family planning clinics. In addition emergency pills are free from NHS Walk-in centres and can be bought from pharmacies by women over 16.

Natural methods

16 It is only possible for your partner to conceive within 24 hours of ovulation. However, because sperm can live for several days, sex that happens up to seven days before ovulation can result in pregnancy (this sex can even be during a period). It is possible to estimate the fertile period by noting certain changes in the body. Using a fertility thermometer and a chart it is possible to detect the sudden rise in temperature of around 0.2 degrees Celsius which occurs at ovulation. Monitoring changes in the cervical mucus helps identify the time before and after ovulation. The mucus becomes thin, watery and clearer before ovulation, and afterwards returns to being thicker, stickier and whiter. When practised according to instruction, natural family planning is said to be 98% effective, although it does take a while to learn it as a method and requires commitment from both partners. Professional advice is essential if you plan to use this method.

Vasectomy (male sterilisation)

17 Vasectomy is a simple and permanent method of contraception. You don't need permission from your partner but obviously it makes good sense. Fortunately there is no reported effect on enjoying sex. The testicles continue to produce sperm but rather than being ejaculated with the semen the sperm are reabsorbed in each testicle. Sperm therefore doesn't build up inside the testicles. As with any surgical procedure you will have to sign a consent form.

18 Although there is no lower age limit for vasectomy, young, childless men need to consider this method carefully to avoid later regret. It should therefore only be chosen by men who, for whatever reason, are sure that they do not want children in the future. Counselling is recommended so that other contraception options can be discussed and the procedure fully understood. A vasectomy immediately following a birth, miscarriage, abortion or family or relationship crisis is a usually a bad idea.

19 You can ask for a general anaesthetic but it is generally performed under a local anaesthetic. A small section of each vas deferens – the tubes carrying the sperm from the testes – is removed through small cuts on either side of the scrotum. The ends of the tubes are then cut or blocked. Stitches are rarely required on the scrotum. It is a simple and safe operation lasting around 10-15 minutes, and can be done in a clinic, hospital outpatient department or doctor's surgery.

20 Discomfort and swelling lasting for a few days is normal but this settles quickly with no other problems. Simple pain-killers help. Occasionally this can last longer and needs your doctor's attention. Strenuous activity should be avoided for a week but you can return to work immediately and have sex as soon as it is comfortable. As the testicles continue to produce testosterone your feelings, sex drive, ability to have an erection and climax won't be affected. Despite numerous scares in the popular media, there are no known long-term risks from a vasectomy.

21 After a vasectomy it can take a few months for all the sperm to disappear from your semen. You need to use another method of contraception until you have had two consecutive semen tests which show that you have no sperm. While vasectomy is highly effective failures are still possible (1 in 2000). The failure rate should be discussed before the operation and it should be pointed out on the consent form. While vasectomy is excellent in preventing pregnancy it will not protect against sexually-transmitted infections. Using a condom is the best protection for this.

22 Reversal operations are possible but not always successful and will depend upon how and when the vasectomy was done. Reversals are not easily available either privately or on the NHS.

Further information

23 If you would like to know more, look in the Contacts section at the back of the book, or contact:
Sexual Health Direct (run by The Family Planning Association)
Tel 0845 310 1334
Mon-Fri 9am-7pm
Website: www.fpa.org.uk

7 Sexually Transmitted Infections (STIs)

1 Sexually transmitted infections (STIs) can infect at any age, whether straight or gay, in a long-term relationship or with a casual partner. Symptoms don't always show up immediately, so the infection could be recent or from a long time ago. It is important always practise safe sex by using a condom. A confidential check-up, and treatment if needed, is available at a genitourinary medicine (GUM) or STI clinic. Call NHS Direct for details of your nearest clinic.

2 GPs and local GUM clinics, which are located at major hospitals, will diagnose and treat such infections. Confidentiality is all-important at these clinics. While honesty to the doctor who asks the questions is obviously vital, as it can be impossible to work out what is wrong without the correct information, a false name or even a number can be used to remain anonymous, although this really is not necessary as these clinics take your confidentiality very seriously. There is no chance of the fact of attendance going any further, even to a GP, let alone any diagnosis that may be made.

3 Certain tests may be needed to make an accurate diagnosis, although it may be fairly obvious on a first visit and the treatment may start immediately with no return needed. It is worth remembering that the doctors and nurses who staff these clinics are professionals who see patients as simply a person who, like any other patient, needs treatment.

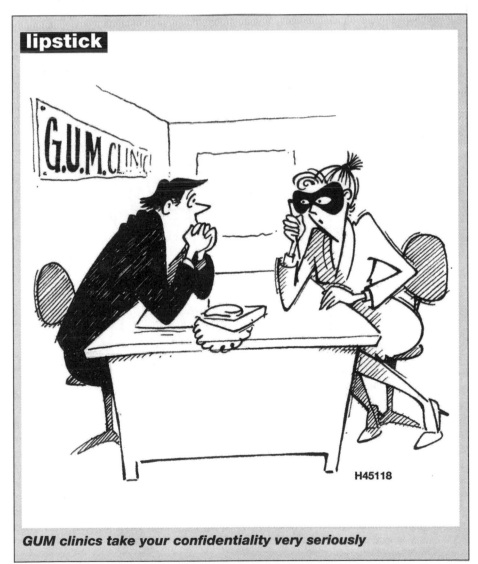

lipstick

G.U.M. CLINIC

H45118

GUM clinics take your confidentiality very seriously

Chlamydia

4 Non-specific urethritis, which simply means an inflammation or infection of the urethra, is an all-embracing term which includes infection by chlamydia. Men and women suffering from this infection may complain of an intense burning sensation when passing water. There may also be a white discharge. It actually causes few problems for men other than this discomfort but can be disastrous if it is passed on to women. Although it is often free of symptoms in women, it is also not only the single biggest cause of infection of the fallopian tubes (pelvic inflammatory disease), leading to infertility and ectopic pregnancy (a potentially lethal condition where the baby attaches to the wall of the fallopian tube instead of the wall of the womb), but can cause blindness and pneumonia in a child born to an infected woman. Condoms provide almost total protection.

5 Chlamydia is treatable with antibiotics but the treatment of female infertility can be complex (see *Infertility*).

Hepatitis B

6 Although Hepatitis B is one of the more deadly sexually transmitted diseases, there is now a protective vaccine to prevent it. Even so, the number of infected people is rising steadily and stands at roughly 700 women each year. It can cause as little as a flu-like illness or as much as total destruction of the liver. Typically, it will cause varying degrees of jaundice (yellowing of the skin and the whites of the eyes). This is caused by the build-up of a pigment which is normally broken down by the liver.

7 Obviously, most people will not require immunisation, but depending upon lifestyle it may be wise to consult a doctor. It is transmitted in the same way as HIV, ie, via bodily fluids. It only requires a tiny fraction of a drop of blood to transmit the disease. For this reason it can be caught from sharing a toothbrush or kissing when there is bleeding from the gums. Worse still, the virus can survive a week or more in the dried state and so can be picked up from, for instance, a razor. There is no way of knowing if the person with whom you are having sex harbours the infection. The

6

incubation period, i.e., how long it takes before the illness manifests itself, is six months from infection. Some people can carry the virus and yet not exhibit the condition.

Genital Herpes

8 This is the third most common STI. Roughly 50% of people who have had one attack never have another. Unfortunately, it is impossible to completely get rid of the virus. Herpes Simplex Virus (HSV) comes in two forms, HSV I and HSV II. Both infect the same places and are likely to infect parts of the body where two types of skin meet together. Both forms can infect the corners of the mouth, the outer parts of the genital areas and even the anus. Both cause crusted blisters and then ulcers that weep a thin, watery substance. This substance is highly infectious, since it contains the virus that causes the condition. Coming in attacks which can last for months and then disappear for years, or even never return, the presence of the sores is a very good sign of being infectious. Even when sores are not present, it might be possible to pass on the infection. Stress and coincidental illness can bring on these attacks. For some women, the condition will pass unnoticed, with only tiny ulcers on the labia (vaginal lips) to show its presence.

9 Anti-viral drugs can be applied directly to the affected skin or taken orally. They are most effective if used before the sores break out. This is signalled by a tingling, itchy, painful sensation in the affected area. They are only effective during the first attack in some people and have not been shown to have any impact on subsequent attacks. Condoms with a spermicide appear to offer greater protection than those without. Condoms give maximum protection.

Genital warts

10 Papilloma viruses, which cause warts, can affect any part of the skin. The virus can be transmitted by physical contact including sexual intercourse. Like the warts commonly seen on people's hands, they can vary in size from tiny skin tags to large fungating masses like cauliflowers. While the latter are hard to miss, the less obvious form can be prevented from causing infection only by covering the area completely. One in eight people attending GUM clinics has genital warts. Around 100,000 people are treated for these warts each year in the UK, many more may simply put up with them, and many people do not even know they have them. It may be a factor in causing cervical cancer in women (see *Cancer of the cervix*).

11 There are drugs which can be applied directly to warts which will cause them to disappear. Liquid nitrogen is now used less often as it can leave a painful 'burn' in such sensitive areas. Genital warts usually cause little discomfort, although they are often itchy and may bleed with scratching. Use a condom to prevent catching them in the first place.

Syphilis

12 A potentially serious condition, syphilis which was almost extinct, is on the big increase in the UK. It is caused by a spirochete, a microscopic parasite, which is highly infectious. Most people are unaware of the infection but if it is not treated it can develop over a number of years into a condition which can affect the brain. Women show few signs of the infection in the early stages except for small ulcers around the vagina so it can go unnoticed by the woman or by their partner during intercourse. The parasite cannot pass through a condom, so this will give almost 100% protection.

13 Penicillin that is given as a single large dose can be given by injection to any part of the body and will invariably cure the condition if it is caught in the early stages.

Trichomoniasis

14 Causing a green discharge from the vagina, this microscopic parasite lives in the urinary tract and usually causes pain when passing water but can be completely symptomless. When it has no effect on the male partner but the female partner complains of a smelly green discharge from the vagina, tests may show its presence in the man.

15 Metronidazole (an antibiotic) is highly effective but must not be taken with alcohol as it can cause severe sickness.

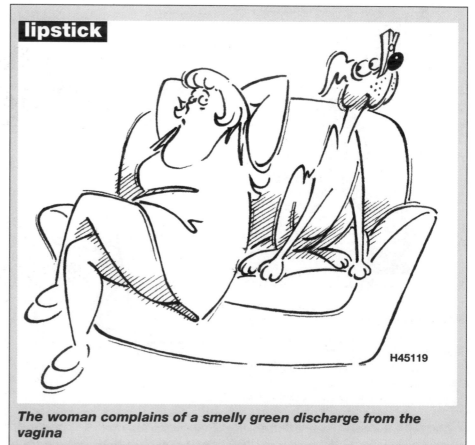

lipstick

H45119

The woman complains of a smelly green discharge from the vagina

Gonorrhoea

16 Caused by a bacterium, this disease is commonly misdiagnosed as it can often give only minimum symptoms. It is commonly known as the clap from the French word *clapoir* meaning sexual sore. Gonorrhoea is not rare. It can cause a yellow/white discharge from the penis and vagina, along with pain on passing water. When infecting the anus there can be a similar discharge. Most of the symptoms will start within 5 days of infection and include a vague ache of the joints and muscles. Although these can disappear after a further 10 or so days, the person remains infectious. It can cause reduced fertility if not treated.

17 Antibiotics are usually effective. Condoms provide almost 100% protection from infection.

HIV & AIDS

18 See Chapter 4.

8 Thrush

1 Candida albicans is a fungus which should not normally be present in large numbers in the vagina. For various reasons it can grow rapidly and cause thrush.

Symptoms

- A creamy thick white vaginal discharge.
- Itchiness and irritation.
- Pain or burning after passing water.

Causes

- A prolonged course of antibiotics.
- The oral contraceptive pill.
- Hormonal changes preceding the period.
- Steroid treatment.
- Diabetes.
- Immune system problems.
- Sexual intercourse with an infected man.

Prevention

- After being on the toilet, wipe from front to back.
- Change underwear frequently, particularly after exercise.
- Choose cotton rather than nylon pants.
- Avoid harsh soaps, they kill the good bacteria which prevent thrush.

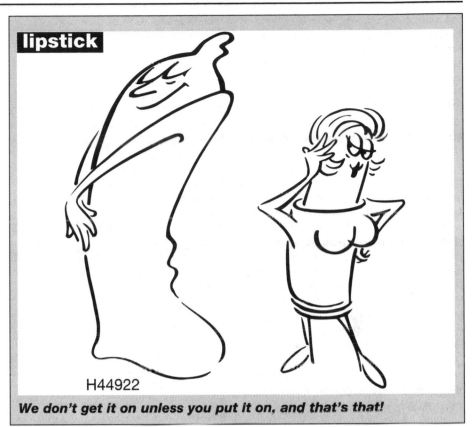

We don't get it on unless you put it on, and that's that!

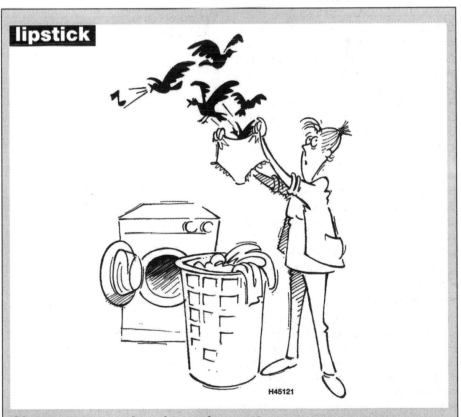

Choose cotton rather than nylon pants

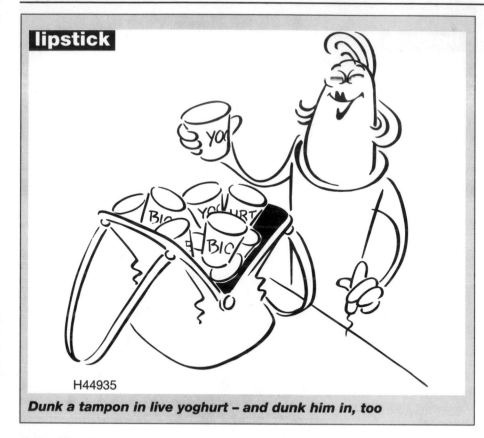

H44935

Dunk a tampon in live yoghurt – and dunk him in, too

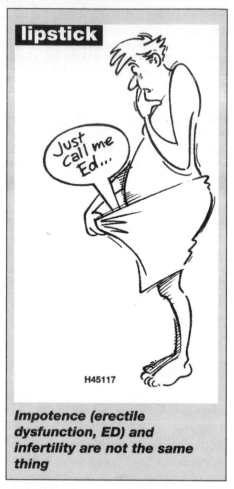

H45117

Impotence (erectile dysfunction, ED) and infertility are not the same thing

Complications

2 Thankfully there are few serious complications of thrush. It can, however, make life very miserable. Sex is painful, as is passing water.

Self care

• Eat live yoghurt and apply it to the vaginal area. It will replace the missing Lactobacillus which prevents thrush.
• Ask the pharmacist for anti-fungal preparations.
• Treat both of you at the same time.

See the doctor if:

• Thrush keeps coming back for no apparent reason
• The discharge changes in smell or appearance
• There is any abdominal pain.

9 Infertility and artificial insemination

1 Fertility problems in men and women can be due to sexually transmitted infections, particularly chlamydia or other forms of pelvic inflammatory disease (PID). These often produce no symptoms so either you or your partner could have an infection without knowing. If you are worried that you may have caught a sexually transmitted infection either recently or in the past, go to a genitourinary medicine (GUM) clinic or sexual health clinic. The service is completely free and confidential. Most large hospitals have a GUM clinic and the Family Planning Association (FPA) can tell you where your nearest one is.

2 Although the term artificial insemination sounds daunting and cold it is actually a simple way of becoming pregnant if it is very difficult or impossible to manage it through sexual intercourse when there is a medical problem preventing conception. Impotence (erectile dysfunction, ED) and infertility are not the same thing. A man can be unable to have an erection yet be perfectly capable of having children by treating the erectile dysfunction or by using assisted methods of conception. Sub-fertility where there are too few sperm in the semen or they are not able to swim correctly does not necessarily mean that you and your partner cannot have children.

3 In cases of ED seminal fluid can often be obtained by masturbation or by massaging the prostate under an anaesthetic. This is called AIP (artificial insemination by partner). With reduced fertility (sub-fertility) pregnancy can sometimes be achieved by placing the semen directly into the cervix. With severely reduced fertility semen can be provided by another man. Most donors remain anonymous although the law is being pressed on this issue should your child wish to know their 'natural' father. This is called AID (artificial insemination by donor). You need to discuss this fully with your partner and medical staff. Of course any form of artificial insemination carries connotations and must always be second best but it is relatively easy, quick and results in the vast majority of cases in a perfectly normal baby. This is the main point to remember when discussing these matters.

How it is performed

4 Ovulation usually occurs 14 days before the start of the next menstrual period so this is the most fertile time and preferable for the procedure. If your partner has regular periods, this point can be known with reasonable accuracy. Ovulation can also sometimes be detected by a half-degree drop in body temperature and by a change in the degree of stickiness of the mucus on the cervix. There are self test kits to determine this most fertile time available from your pharmacist or family planning clinics.

5 Semen is inserted using a syringe high into the vagina or possibly into the opening of the womb (uterus) at the cervix. So long as there is no medical condition preventing conception there is a high probability of conception. You can perform this yourselves or it can be performed in a fertility clinic.

Results

6 All pregnancies are followed by careful monitoring through ultrasound and possibly amniocentesis so the chances of an abnormal birth are low. For most couples the birth of a perfectly normal baby helps overcome any of the residual emotional distress caused by the procedure.

Self Help

7 There are some things you and your partner can do to help you be fit and healthy for pregnancy. Rubella infection in pregnancy can harm a developing baby so your partner should have a Rubella (German Measles) test to check if she is immune and if she needs a vaccination.

8 All women planning a baby should take 400 micrograms (0.4mg) of folic acid every day from the time they stop using contraception until the twelfth week of pregnancy, as folic acid reduces the risk of a baby having neural tube defects, such as spina bifida. You can get folic acid from pharmacies.

9 Eat a balanced diet and try to eat five portions of fruit and vegetables a day. Don't eat too many foods that contain a lot of fat or sugar.

10 Both you and your partner should try to give smoking up before as smoking is known to carry risks for the developing baby and also to newborn babies. This is important for men as smokers tend to produce fewer sperm and have more damaged sperm.

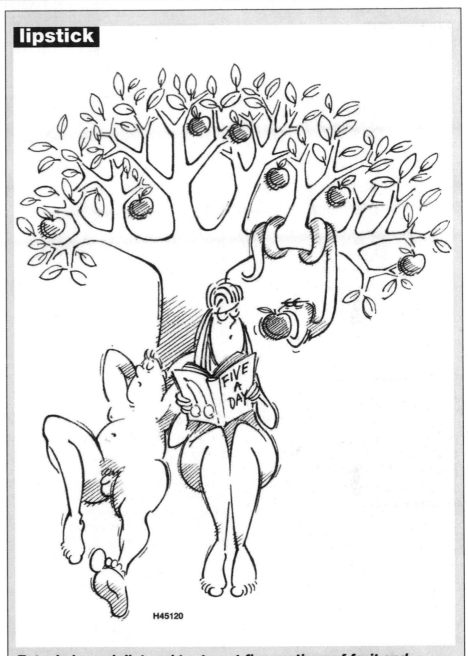

lipstick

H45120

Eat a balanced diet and try to eat five portions of fruit and vegetables a day

11 You may need to reduce the amount of alcohol you drink – phone NHS Direct or ask your pharmacist for advice.

12 Weight can affect the way your partner produces eggs – ovulation – so women who are very underweight or overweight might want to talk to NHS Direct or their practice nurse.

Counselling and support

13 Many couples feel that the many hospital visits needed and the time spent waiting between treatments to learn if each stage has worked is stressful. All units providing IVF and other licensed conception techniques offer counselling which allows you both to talk through what the treatment entails and how you feel about it, and can give support during the process and if the treatment fails.

14 If you don't want to see a counsellor at the clinic you are attending, the British Infertility Counsellors Association can put you in touch with your nearest

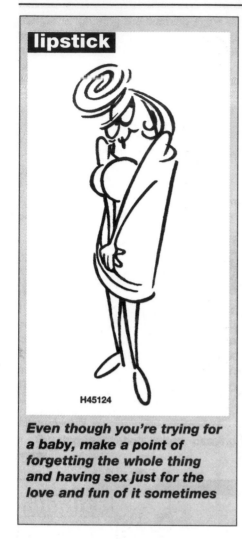

lipstick

Even though you're trying for a baby, make a point of forgetting the whole thing and having sex just for the love and fun of it sometimes

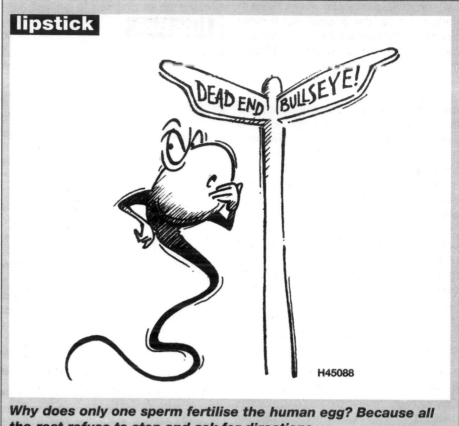

lipstick

Why does only one sperm fertilise the human egg? Because all the rest refuse to stop and ask for directions

infertility counsellor. Some people find being in contact with others in a similar situation or with a support group helps them through infertility. You can contact CHILD, The National Fertility Support Network or ISSUE, The National Fertility Association for details of your nearest one.

10 Cancer of the ovaries

See Chapter 7.

11 The bloke's guide to pregnancy

Us men hate to ask for help but things could be better for everyone if we devoted as much time to understanding the mysteries of pregnancy as we do to understanding the conundrum of how the toilet seat is always down again next time we go to the bathroom.

Men are under increasing pressure to be more empathic during pregnancy and labour. Even Bill Crosby realised the importance of seeing things from the woman's perspective. When asked was labour painful he answered, 'It sure is. She damn near squeezed the fingers right off me'. In truth, it is a joint decision between partners just how much the man should get involved. But a bit more insight makes the decision more informed and less of a knee jerk reaction.

Having a baby is more exciting than your team winning (honest)

1 Not all men are ecstatic on hearing the good news and there are invariably mixed emotions. Tearing all your hair out and ripping up your season ticket to Manchester United will not go down well. A bottle of champagne (of which you will be able to drink the greater part quite legitimately) most definitely will in all senses of the word.

2 Your partner will be offered a choice of ways in which she can have antenatal care. This will be influenced by her previous pregnancies, medical health and social factors such as living in a remote part of the country which only the flying doctor can get to in a rush. No matter what anyone tells you, being pregnant is not an illness and having babies may occasionally be a tad tricky but it is still normal and women have been doing it for a very long time. Women in their first pregnancy where there is some reason to want closer observation, or if a previous pregnancy was difficult, are often advised full hospital care. A named consultant and a named midwife will take responsibility for your partner's checks as she approaches her delivery dates. Parental classes are usually held in the same department, which is just great for ensuring as few men attend as possible. Pity, as they are great fun especially for us fat dads who empathise so much better. You are welcome to come along to these antenatal sessions, especially for the first ultrasound scan. Never underestimate how scared your partner can be at that first session. A hot sweaty hand in her hotter sweatier hand helps more than you will know. It's easy to forget in that darkened room with the glowing, totally incomprehensible screen that abnormalities are rare and all unusual positions in the womb can be safely dealt with.

3   Most GPs will offer a mix of checks at their surgery along with visits to the maternity hospital. Convenient and quick, it also ensures contact with a doctor who generally knows a lot about your partner's medical history. You can also attend these just like the hospital sessions. However, I have yet to find men beating a path to my door which is not surprising as most will only attend the surgery when they are in the terminal stages of a condition or Liverpool FC are playing Manchester United mid-week.

Early days, happy returns

4   Morning sickness baffles most men. Chundering after 10 pints and a curry is perfectly reasonable behaviour but to wake up with pursed lips and wide expectant eyes is patently odd. This can be so bad, especially in the first two semesters (6 months) women sometimes dehydrate, lose weight and need to be admitted to hospital. There is probably nothing you can do when it gets this bad but for the less traumatic versions many women find tricks to reduce the sickness. A small dry biscuit with a cup of tea or milk is a common strategy but it only works if it is there *when she first awakes.* Five minutes too late and your pillow has a permanent stilton flavour.

Two to tango

5   When it comes to making babies Aristotle had a theory. The woman provided the canvas while the man supplied the paint. This is a pretty good reflection of male dominance in the medical profession. Housework can be a bit like that too. Supplying the canvas can be pretty hard work, not least because your weight is steadily increasing, pressure is building up on your diaphragm, bladder and digestive system and most importantly, your hormones are doing a samba with your emotions.

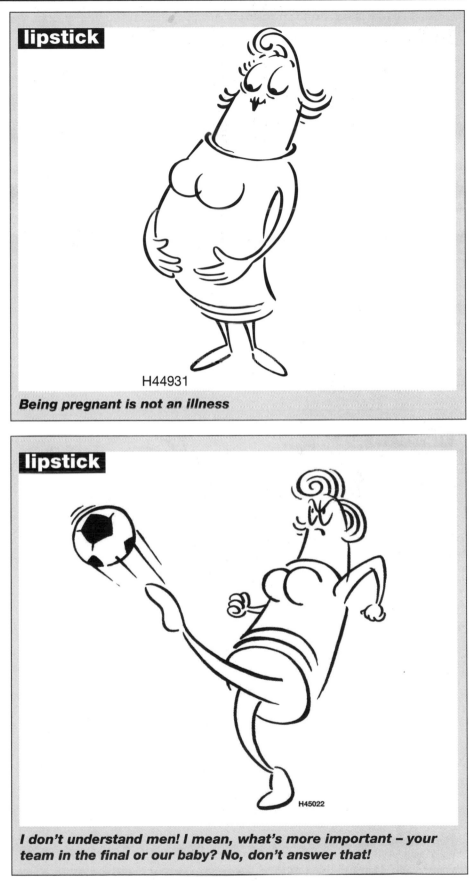

lipstick

H44931

Being pregnant is not an illness

lipstick

H45022

I don't understand men! I mean, what's more important – your team in the final or our baby? No, don't answer that!

6

6 Being heavier is not just the problem, it's being heavier just in one place, the front. This puts strain on the back muscles so bending over or simply standing up straight, gets increasingly difficult. Watching out for when she has something to pick up and darting in like Sir Walter Raleigh, giving a back massage during the day as well as at night and more to the point, doing the housework all make for better tangos, if not sambas. You and I know that constant childcare is at best challenging and, at worst, a weapon of man's destruction. Picking them up on your foot, being the horse or giving great piggy back rides is fine so long as there is someone else to finish the job off. Now is the time to do the feeding and toileting as well.

Natural but nasty

7 Be prepared for fire in the hole. Heartburn is common during pregnancy not least because of the pressure on the stomach. Your kind offer to cook all the meals will be less gratefully received if vindaloo, chilli con carne and deep fried Mars Bars are the only things on the menu. Smaller, frequent, more easily digested meals on the other hand will be deeply and more permanently appreciated. You may also find your own sleep less disturbed by two or more concurrent people diving for the antacids every night. A nocturnal glass of ice cold milk on hand anyway makes for similar affection. Your stainless steel fishing vacuum flask has found a new and probably more productive use.

Great training

8 Getting up in the middle of the night is par for the course when having kids. So your partner's frequent excursion to the loo (pressure on the bladder), constant shifting in the bed (pressure on the pointy bits) and irrational demands for a life-saving Belgian chocolate at 3 am (hormone shifts) should be seen as great training. Leave the light on in the loo, buy a better mattress, give great massage and work out the shortest route to the all-night delicatessen. Toughens you up, boy, for the big push to come later. Sudden, swift and severe shifts in mood are also part of the equation as hormones loop around like demented jugglers. Expect weeping followed by ecstatic laughter at banal baby-product adverts. Join in. Has to be better than a party political broadcast. Now is the time for being Nelson Mandela not George Bush. Just because she can't explain why the bedroom has to be painted pink, the baby cot erected from a flat pack, the stairs cordoned off like East Berlin at 1 am *six months before the baby is even due* is perfectly reasonable to her. Think of it this way, if a man says something in a forest and no woman hears him say it, is he still wrong? Exactly.

9 You are going to have an interesting nine months with a finale that throws the Cup Final into a cocked hat *and* you will be on the winning side. Good luck dad.

12 Confirmation of pregnancy

1 Testing for pregnancy used to involve rabbits. Things have progressed and now most of the tests for early pregnancy depend on the presence of chorionic gonadotrophin. This hormone is first present in the blood, but soon afterwards appears in the urine. A simple dipstick test into fresh morning urine can detect pregnancy with about a 98% certainty. As they say, you can't be a little bit pregnant.

2 While kits for performing these tests are available over-the-counter from pharmacies, there are even more sensitive immunological tests to detect the hormone by its combination with pre-prepared specific antibodies to it which can confirm pregnancy within a week of conception. These are normally done in a hospital laboratory. If these tests are positive the accuracy is nearly 100% certain; if the test is negative, about 80% certain.

3 Missing one or more periods in a healthy woman of child bearing age can result from certain medical conditions but pregnancy is probably the most common cause. Many women can tell if they are pregnant even before they have had a test performed or have missed a period.

lipstick

I've always liked pickles on my ice cream! How could you eat the last one?

H45021

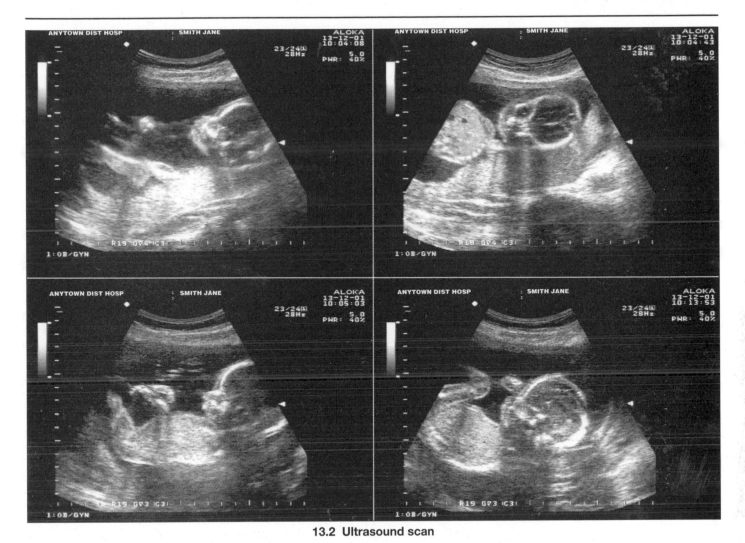

13.2 Ultrasound scan

13 Ultrasound

1 Incredible advances have taken place over the past 40 years when it comes to monitoring the development of the unborn baby. Ultrasound scanning has become increasingly important as a way of scanning without using any radiation such as X-rays.

How it is done

2 A beam of 'sound' at a frequency of about three to ten million cycles per second is sent into the abdomen above the uterus using a machine which looks like a hand held scanner used for computers. Tissues of different density produce echoes which return to the machine. In this way a picture of the inside of the body can be created. To make sure there is good contact with the device producing the ultrasound waves, a special gel is applied to the region to be examined. This can be a bit cold but is completely harmless. It once took considerable training to interpret the pictures produced but they are now so clear the mum and dad can see for themselves. This can spoil the element of surprise when it come to the sex of the baby and you may be advised to 'look away' while the result is shown if you still want the mystery to remain.

Complications

3 So far as is known, ultrasound of the intensity and frequency used in scanning, is completely harmless. Millions of pregnant women, and their babies, have had scans with no harm. You must balance the perception of danger from scanning against the consequences of an undetected serious malformation.

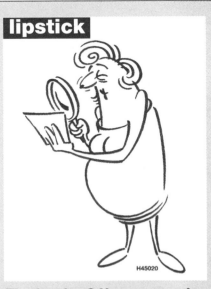

lipstick

H45020

That's a boy? Hmmm, need a microscope. Takes after his dad, doesn't he?

6

Uses of Ultrasound

4 Without doubt the main advantage of routine ultrasound screening is the early detection and management of foetal abnormalities.

5 Ultrasound is extensively used in obstetrics mainly because of the possible danger of X-rays to the developing baby. Most pregnant women are screened by ultrasound, usually around the 16th to 20th week of pregnancy. Ultrasound has many uses in maternity units. It can:

• Detect twins.

• Display the position of the afterbirth (placenta) so problems arising from abnormal position, such as placenta praevia (where the placenta is blocking the 'way out' for the baby) can be managed.

• Facilitate amniocentesis, foetal blood sampling, chorionic villus sampling and foetoscopy.

• Confirm that the baby is of a size appropriate to the stage of pregnancy.

• Detect major foetal abnormalities such as anencephaly (poor brain development) and spina bifida (a lack of bone covering parts of the spinal cord).

• Measure the rates of blood flow through the heart valves and the large arteries of the baby's heart.

• Sometimes detect certain forms of congenital heart disease.

6 Under ultrasound control, foetal blood samples can be obtained through a fine tube, and analysed to detect coagulation disorders, infections, haemoglobin abnormalities and immunodeficiency disorders.

7 Ultrasound enables the taking of biopsies (small samples of tissue). Blood transfusion in rhesus disease can be done while the baby is still in the womb, drug treatment given, and even certain forms of surgery can be performed guided by ultrasound.

14 Ectopic pregnancy

1 Thankfully the vast majority of pregnancies are uneventful and have happy endings. Unfortunately the increasing number of women infected with chlamydia is shadowed by a rise in a dangerous complication of pregnancy where the fertilized egg (ovum) becomes implanted in an abnormal site inside the body instead of in the womb lining. The great majority of these ectopic pregnancies, over 95%, occur in a fallopian tube connecting the ovaries to the womb.

2 There has been a large increase in ectopic pregnancies in the last 30 years, from about 4 per 1000 pregnancies in 1970 to about 20 per 1000. Chlamydia, a sexually transmitted infection is a major factor as there has been a corresponding increase in infection of this bacterium which causes pelvic inflammatory disease (PID) leading to inflammation and narrowing of the fallopian tubes.

3 Early diagnosis of ectopic pregnancy is vital as it can cause severe internal bleeding, further damage to the fallopian tubes not to mention endangering the life of the woman.

Symptoms

4 The symptoms of ectopic pregnancy can mimic an appendicitis but usually start with cramping period-like pains and slight vaginal bleeding occurring soon after the first missed period.

Causes

5 Around half of all women operated on for ectopic pregnancy have evidence of pelvic inflammatory disease the basic cause of which is often Chlamydial infection.

Diagnosis

6 Ultrasound scanning has improved the speedy and accurate diagnosis of an ectopic pregnancy, vital if further damage to the woman's reproductive system is to be avoided. This is often followed by direct examination through a viewing tube passed through a small opening in the wall of the abdomen (laparoscopy). Suspicion is raised in the first place by the symptoms and a positive pregnancy test.

7 If she has pains and feels something is wrong, don't ignore it; support her in seeking help at once.

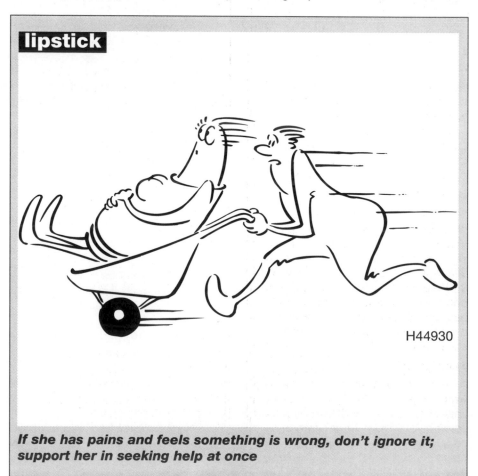

lipstick

H44930

If she has pains and feels something is wrong, don't ignore it; support her in seeking help at once

Prevention

8 It is impossible to prevent an ectopic pregnancy other than by using safer sex (condoms) which give almost 100% protection from chlamydia infection, the single greatest cause.

Complications

9 Thanks to swift medical care relatively few women will die from an ectopic pregnancy but it leaves scars not just on the fallopian tube which further reduce the chance of a successful pregnancy but also on her abdomen and possibly her mind. Loss of any baby is bad enough but many women are deeply worried by the thought of future pregnancy.

Treatment

10 The woman must be brought to A&E as soon as possible. Treatment is by urgent operation to remove the growing embryo. This is mainly done by laparoscopic surgery.

15 Pre-eclampsia

1 Memories are fading over the impact this condition had over the lives of women and their unborn child. Once the scourge of pregnancy, pre-eclampsia is now not only rare but also treatable when caught early. It is a disorder originating in the placenta that, once under way, can cause severe damage to the circulatory system of both mother and baby.

Diagnosis

2 A sudden and rapid rise in the blood pressure and the presence of the protein albumin in the urine are the two major signs of pre-eclampsia, both of which can be detected by a GP or midwife.

3 Pregnancy is not an illness and you don't have to treat her like an invalid – but encourage her to attend all the check-ups and see her doctor ASAP if she feels unwell.

Treatment

4 Survival for both mother and child was once rare. Now bed rest is an important measure but established pre-eclampsia needs urgent treatment to sedate the mother, get the blood pressure down and deliver the baby as soon as possible.

16 Maternal Rubella

See Chapter 2.

17 Miscarriage

1 Losing the baby before the 28th week of pregnancy is called a spontaneous miscarriage and occurs most commonly during the first three months of pregnancy.

2 It is unfortunately more common than most men think. There is still a reluctance to discuss these things openly. At least one pregnancy in ten ends in miscarriage, most of these occurring at an early stage. In many of these cases, the woman concerned is never aware that she is pregnant and experiences a late, and perhaps unusually severe, period.

Signs of miscarriage

3 Recognising that something has gone wrong is not always easy and people can make mistakes in both directions. Any pain in the abdomen, particularly if it is associated with blood loss from the vagina, needs to be investigated. Simply a lack of movement or just a feeling that something is wrong can be a sign. Many relatively minor conditions can mimic these symptoms. Urinary tract infections (cystitis) can often cause abdominal pain and even some blood in the urine. Even the pain of constipation has been mistaken for the onset of a miscarriage. More obvious and severe lower abdominal pain suggests a possible pregnancy outside the womb (ectopic pregnancy).

Causes

4 In the vast majority of cases there will be no obvious cause but there are some well recognised factors such as:
- An ectopic (see *Ectopic pregnancy*) or unsuitable site in the womb for the baby to develop normally.
- An abnormality inside the womb.
- Instability of the neck of the womb which may open too soon (incompetent cervix). This affects about one pregnancy in a hundred and causes repeated,

painless, spontaneous miscarriages around the fourth or fifth month of pregnancy.
- Any hormone imbalance which affects the pregnancy.
- A GU (genito urinary) infection.

Prevention

5 Miscarriage from incompetent cervix can often be avoided by inserting a temporary encircling stitch (a Shirodkar suture).

Treatment

6 If the miscarriage is missed or incomplete a minor operation, under general anaesthesia, may be needed. Suction is used to clear the womb, and the lining is carefully scraped with a sharp-edged spoon called a curette. A drug is then given to cause the womb to contract, and antibiotics may also be necessary. The woman is usually able to go home the next day.

7 Miscarriage later in pregnancy is less common and is often associated with abnormalities of the womb or with inability of the cervix to remain closed (cervical incompetence). Full gynaecological investigation will reveal the cause of this in about 40% of cases. Support from yourself along with good medical advice is needed. Generally she will be scanned by ultrasound (a painless, harmless, examination using sound waves which pass though skin to produce a picture of the baby) and the baby examined for its well-being.

8 Relatives may mistakenly try to be positive with comments such as "there must have been something wrong with the baby" or "you can always try again". What is forgotten is that you and your partner are already grieving. While it is true that major abnormalities can lead to loss of the baby, we still know precious little about the process of miscarriage and why apparently perfectly normal pregnancies come to an early end. Suggesting to your partner that she may have produced an abnormal baby will not help for the next pregnancy. You should recognise her need to grieve and to supply emotional support accordingly. Unfortunately, people may forget your own suffering. You too will be grieving but people may not realise. This is particularly true when there have been a number of miscarriages or if you have

6

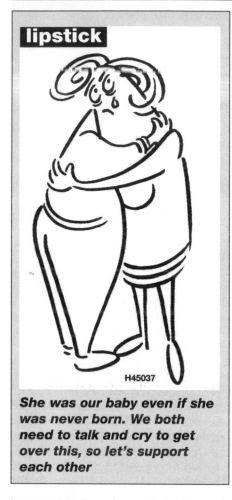

lipstick

H45037

She was our baby even if she was never born. We both need to talk and cry to get over this, so let's support each other

lipstick

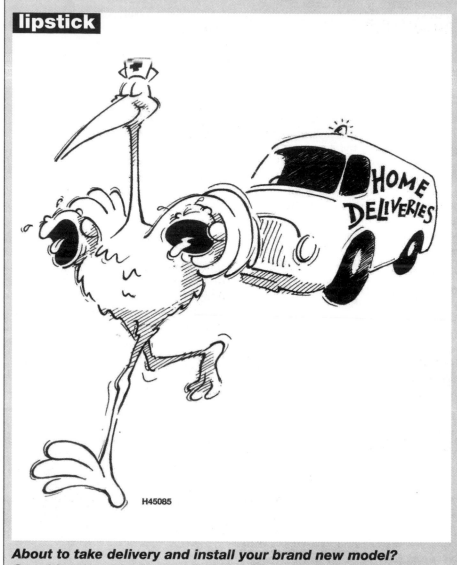

H45085

About to take delivery and install your brand new model? Consider the old adage, 'when you have tried everything else, read the instruction manual'

been trying for a long time. It's worth remembering that part of the process of grieving is to strike out at those closest to them so be prepared for misdirected anger and frustration. There are counsellors available for men as well as women and the maternity unit will put you in touch with them.

18 The Big Push

1 Remember this word – 'contractions' – practise saying it a few times. You are going to hear this word a great deal and it has nothing to do with binding agreements. Messrs Braxton & Hicks have a lot to answer for. Their name goes with lazy drawn out occasional contractions getting progressively stronger and more frequent as pregnancy progresses. Unfortunately they are also perennially confused with the onset of labour. If labour is really

taking place, the contractions began some time, possibly hours, ago. Each contraction will generally be less than twenty minutes apart and last more than forty seconds. There may also be a 'show' of watery mucus from the vagina. No food for your partner from here on, just in case she needs a general anaesthetic.

Labour is working: how true

2 Labour wards are not electoral regions full of spin doctors and thankfully the staff are less likely these days to treat the father as a useless lump of dad, prone to trip over the drip or switch off

the heart monitor instead of the TV. Even so it helps to know what is going on. There are basically three stages of labour. These overlap and vary in time, often considerably, from woman to woman.

The first stage

3 The membrane (amnion) surrounding the baby generally ruptures well into labour and releases the liquid in which the baby floated. This first stage continues until the cervix – opening of the womb – is fully dilated and as most babies know an exit sign when they see one, stick their heads in the doorway.

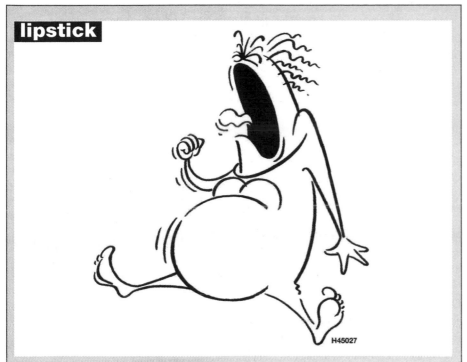

lipstick

Chocolate! I need chocolate! If you felt the way I do, you'd need chocolate!

The second stage

4 Timing is everything. Life is tricky at the best of times without having your head stuck in a very narrow space for an entire episode of Coronation Street. Similarly, a too rapid delivery can be dangerous. Your partner will want to push very hard at this point so it's important to relay her all the instructions from the midwife. Think dipstick not champagne cork. Talking to her, giving encouragement, a cool damp cloth on her forehead along with helping with the gas mixture, makes her job a little easier. Lady-like language tends to go out the door. You might also be thinking a tad more than, 'goodness me, you don't see that every day'.

5 An episiotomy, where the lower part of the vaginal wall is cut as the baby's head appears, is less often performed today but can help prevent severe tearing. Local anaesthetic is always applied first, but it still looks barbaric. It will be later repaired by stitching. It can help if you are there for distraction and provide support. After an injection to

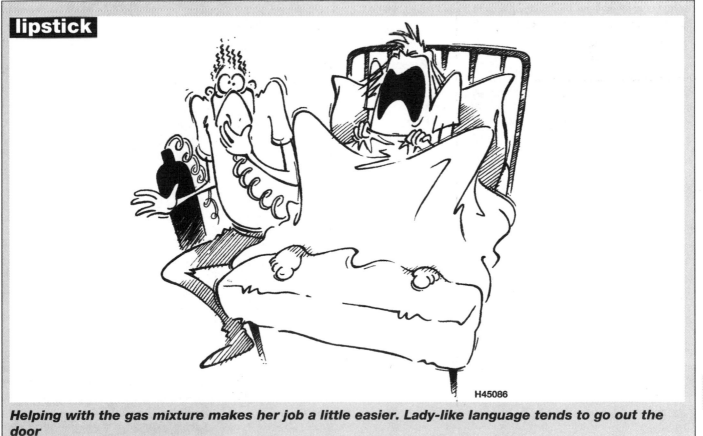

lipstick

Helping with the gas mixture makes her job a little easier. Lady-like language tends to go out the door

6

encourage the womb to contract and expel the placenta – afterbirth – the umbilical cord is cut and sealed at each end. Now you truly share your baby.

The third stage

6 Placentas are surprisingly large organs and you will be forgiven for thinking someone carelessly left a few pounds of tripe lying around. They are carefully examined in this final stage, checking no bits have been left behind causing infection later on.

First impressions

7 Newly born babies are always short of air so they normally appear blue except for a fine white cheesy substance (vernix) covering their bodies. Babies faces and heads usually look distorted, not really surprising after the moulding needed to get through the narrow canal. A few good breaths, a quick rub and they actually look almost human. Not all babies cry when they are born, although it is encouraging as they are obviously expanding their lungs. Squeezing during birth and crying afterwards helps to get rid of the fluid present in their lungs. Few men, no matter how big or tough, can

resist this little bundle when handed to them and contrary to myth never drop them, invariably having the decency to faint afterwards. You might even feel a few contractions yourself, Dad.

19 Stillbirth

1 Few disasters that life throws at you can compare with the birth of a dead baby. Often there is no obvious cause and you both are left with a bewildering mix of emotions. It is confused with miscarriage but is said to occur after 24 weeks of pregnancy. The good news is that the number of stillbirths has fallen steadily during the last 50 years.

Causes

2 Some medical conditions increase the risk: diabetes; high blood pressure in the mother; rhesus incompatibility (blue babies); maternal high blood pressure and seizures in pregnancy (eclampsia); severe malformations; inadequacy of the afterbirth (placenta); or infections such as toxoplasmosis, German measles

(rubella), syphilis or herpes simplex, but often the reason will never be known. It is important to talk to your doctor about future babies as they can often give reassurance that this was a dreadful one-off and that it should not stop you and your partner from having a baby in future. On the other hand they may be able to reduce the risk of it happening again by looking at any medical conditions that could have contributed. Some people will try to be helpful by saying there must have been something wrong with the baby. This simply makes the woman even more worried for the next pregnancy. In truth there is often no reason found for this dreadful thing to happen. Constant support and accepting that bereavement often causes people to lash out at those they love most, is the very best you can do for your partner and your future relationship.

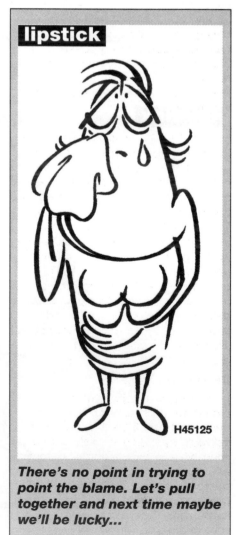

There's no point in trying to point the blame. Let's pull together and next time maybe we'll be lucky...

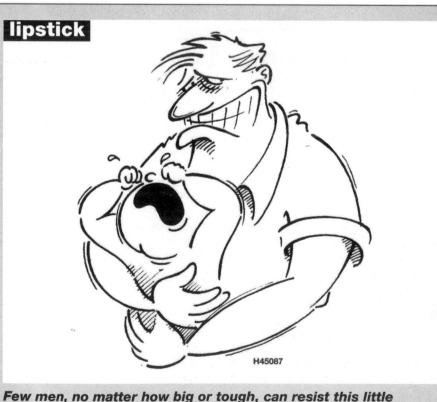

Few men, no matter how big or tough, can resist this little bundle

20 Assisted delivery

1 The reason why many doctors prefer hospital deliveries is that unfortunately not all deliveries go according to plan. Most problems, like a breech birth where the bottom and not the head present first, however, can be predicted by good ante-natal care including the use of ultrasound scans. Should a delivery pose a problem, if the second stage is too prolonged for instance, a number of alternatives can be used depending on the nature of the problem.

Forceps & Ventouse cup

2 Forceps conjure up all kinds of misconceptions. Not only can they save the life of the child but also avoid having to perform a Caesarean section. They are essentially a pair of scoops which fit around the baby's head. Using gentle pulling, the doctor can manoeuvre the baby for a safe delivery. Despite all the old wives tales it is very safe when performed by an expert, although it does look a little dramatic. Ventouse cup is a vacuum assisted delivery where a soft rubber cup is applied over the babies head and a gentle suction applied which keeps the cup in place. the doctor can then manoeuvre the baby through its delivery. Both methods tend to cause some temporary distortion to the babies head either from slight marks of the forceps particularly about the ears or a pronounced cap on the baby's head from the vacuum delivery. Neither is permanent or dangerous. Again it is a balance of safety for the mother and child versus discomfort of the assisted delivery. Supporting your partner is important and many doctors will not only allow you stay with your partner but also prefer you do so.

Caesarean section

3 Part of the reason why modern child birth is so much safer for the mother, is the speed at which the baby can be delivered by an operation should it prove impossible to allow a normal or forceps assisted, delivery. Placenta praevia, where the placenta is either over or very close to the opening of the womb, used to be invariably fatal for both mother and child as there was no way of detecting its

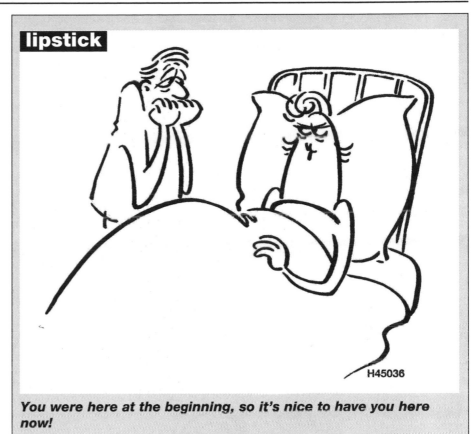

lipstick

H45036

You were here at the beginning, so it's nice to have you here now!

presence until delivery. Few women survived as there was invariably a great deal of blood loss. Thanks to ultrasound examination and Caesarean section, this is rarely the case. The operation can be performed under a general anaesthetic or by freezing the lower part of the body by injecting a local anaesthetic into the area around the lower spinal cord. This latter method allows the mother to see her baby as it is born and is pain free. You will be usually be invited to sit with your partner and is an experience which, like normal child birth, can be usefully shared. Be reassured that you will be protected from the nuts and bolts of the operation allowing you to concentrate on supporting your partner. You will be surprised at the informality of the event with every emphasis being made to allow you and your partner to enjoy your new baby. Most babies will spend a little time in an incubator after a Caesarean delivery as they can need a little more help keeping warm and getting enough air at the beginning.

4 Many women worry about the scar the operation will leave and the effect it could have on any future attempts at having children by a normal delivery. For almost all Caesarean sections the scar will be very low down on the abdomen and runs side ways not up and down the abdomen. It is usually well covered by a pair of bikini bottoms and is often referred to as a bikini incision. While some complications of pregnancy and delivery which require a section may make a normal delivery dangerous, this is by no means true in all cases. It is your understanding of these points and help in the discussion which will reassure your partner when the day comes.

21 Breast feeding

1 Even formula milk manufacturers agree that breast milk is the ideal source of nourishment for the new-born baby as it not only provides the nutritional balance of proteins, sugar and fat, it also prevents gastroenteritis and may even protect the mother from breast cancer.

6

2 As the immune system of the new baby is immature and has not yet had the opportunity to produce antibodies, maternal antibodies to a range of infections can be absorbed by the baby to give a valuable degree of passive immunity. This helps cover the period before its own immune system can take over.

3 Once the placenta has been delivered, the hormone prolactin is released from a gland in the brain, the pituitary, which stimulates the breasts to produce milk. The stimulus of handling and touching the breasts and especially the suckling by the baby increases the production of prolactin and it is essentially this stimulus that maintains the flow.

4 So long as suckling continues, milk will continue to be produced. This is the basis for the 'wet nursing' of former times.

5 Milk production is fully established two to five days after delivery, and the breasts become enlarged by about one third in volume and are usually tender.

6 Most of the actual synthesis of the milk occurs while the baby is suckling and the prolactin levels are at their highest. The milk secreted under the influence of prolactin must move into the ducts behind the nipple before the baby can suck and squeeze it out.

7 This movement into the ducts is called milk let-down and is under the influence of another pituitary hormone called oxytocin. Like prolactin, this hormone is prompted by suckling and by psychological factors. A nursing mother may find that she will leak milk on hearing her baby cry.

8 Although in about 50% of cases breast feeding prevents any eggs being released from the ovaries continued milk production should not be relied upon as a contraceptive. When nursing is discontinued for a few days, the pressure of the milk closes off the small blood vessels in the gland and, since the milk is secreted from the blood, the supply soon fails.

9 Fat cells in the breast connective tissue increase in size and the breasts usually end up larger than before the pregnancy.

10 No formula milk, however expensive, can compare with breast milk, which contains fat, proteins (casein, lactalbumin, lactoglobulin), sugar (lactose), vitamins (C, A and D), minerals (sodium, potassium, calcium, iron, magnesium, etc) but are an essential substitute when breast feeding cannot be performed for whatever reason.

11 Even so for many reasons breast feeding is far from ideal for all women and circumstances alter cases. There is now huge pressure on women which needs to be balanced by personal preference and circumstance.

12 Some women are taking prescription drugs that the baby should not have. There are also some infections that can be passed on in the milk. Careers and breast feeding don't always mix, and many women are shy about feeding in public places.

Breast feeding: All gain, no pain

• Breast feeding protects against gastrointestinal infections.

• Breast feeding protects against respiratory infections.

• Breast feeding protects against urinary tract infections.

• Breast feeding protects against ear infections.

• Breast feeding protects against allergic diseases (eczema, asthma and wheezing).

• Breast feeding can have a protective effect against the development of Type I diabetes.

• Breast feeding is associated with higher scores for cognitive development and intelligence.

• Babies who are breast fed longest grow up to have significantly increased intelligence as adults.

• Breast feeding has a protective effect against childhood cancers.

• Breast feeding is associated with a lower risk of Sudden Infant Death Syndrome (cot death).

• Increased duration of breast feeding is associated with a decline in the prevalence of dental malocclusion (sticking-out teeth).

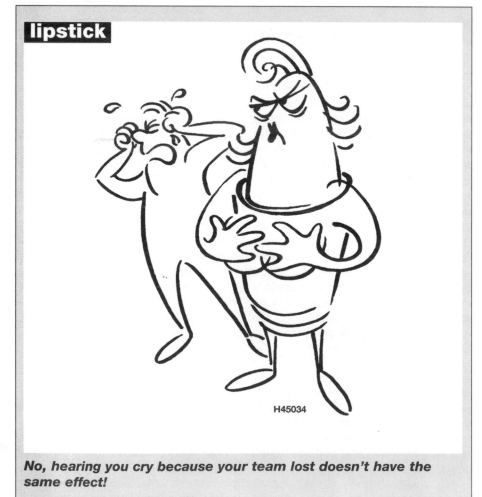

lipstick

H45034

No, hearing you cry because your team lost doesn't have the same effect!

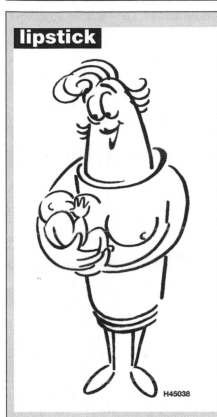

In fact, the only argument against it is that the little blighter sometimes bites, and you get jealous! Support me in feeding our kid – you can have sole rights again later!

13 The benefits to the mothers are also significant.

• A review of 47 breast cancer studies that included information on breast feeding patterns found that the longer women breast fed the more they are protected against breast cancer.

• A multi-national study showed a 20-30 % decrease in the risk of ovarian cancer among women who lactated for at least 2 months per pregnancy compared to those who did not.

• Breast feeding is associated with subsequent higher bone mineral density and lower risk of hip fractures.

22 Breast cancer

See Chapter 7.

23 Menopause

1 Some doctors need to be reminded that menopause is natural not a medical condition. We see a similar approach to pregnancy and childbirth. It is an inevitable consequence of maturity, as the number of eggs released from the ovaries declines so periods become irregular, shorter and eventually cease. There is no 'normal' age for this to happen and can range from 40 years to 58 years. The average age for the menopause is around 51 years. A quarter of women will experience no difference except the lack of periods, half will report mild changes and a further quarter will experience marked changes in the way they feel along with physical differences.

Symptoms

2 Few changes in life come with such variation in impact. There may well be a similar impact on relationships but not all women will experience physical symptoms and the severity will also vary. Even the duration will range from a few months to a few years but the most common are:

• Hot flushes.
• Vaginal dryness.
• Pain on intercourse (mainly due to dryness).
• Sweating.
• Headaches.
• Irregular heart beats.
• Joint pain.

3 As with physical symptoms, the non-physical changes also vary greatly between women but include:

• Irritability.
• Depression.
• Tiredness.
• Poor concentration.

4 These can all lead to a lack of confidence, worries over the future, poor sleep patterns and strains on relationships.

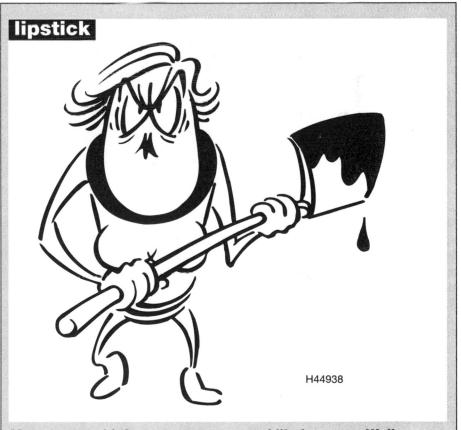

My partner said the menopause never killed anyone. Well, you could have fooled me!

6

Causes

5 Menopause is normal but that doesn't mean that like many things with aging we can't make life better. The changes in hormonal states, particularly the drop in oestrogen levels, are the biggest factors but simply recognising these changes are as important as trying to interfere with natural hormone levels.

Prevention

6 Menopause is a phenomenon as old as women so it is not surprising there are 'natural' treatments such as plant phyto-oestrogens which are said to act in a similar way to hormone replacement therapy (HRT). HRT itself has pros and cons - see *Hormone replacement therapy* in Chapter 2.

7 Whether or not your partner opts for HRT, she is still entitled to have her symptoms taken seriously by you and by her GP. Other than HRT, there are specific treatments for some unpleasant symptoms.

Complications

8 The most important medical complication is osteoporosis (see *Osteoporosis*) or bone thinning. Vaginal bleeding, no matter how small, should be reported to the doctor if it occurs after the menopause has settled as cancer of the womb can occur even after menopause.

Self care

9 Regular activity is valuable in maintaining muscle tone and beating depression, especially any activity such as walking or cycling causing slight breathlessness.
• Even 15 minutes per day will make a disproportionate difference.

• Vaginal lubricants will improve your love making but remember to use water based lubricants if you or your partner are using condoms.
• Continue to use contraception for 2 years after the last period if it ended while she was under 50 years old. Otherwise use contraception for 1 year.
• You may find her hot flushes are triggered by certain drinks. Night sweats thankfully decline but a change of tops and nightwear at hand can help.

10 Menopause no longer makes pregnancy an impossibility. There are medical treatments which can allow a normal pregnancy for women in their 60s and onwards. The raging debate over this seems to ignore the common phenomenon of older men having children late in life.

Chapter 7
Pass the MoT (avoiding cancer)

Contents

1 Introduction

Cancer is common and because we are generally living longer it's becoming commoner. Although no one would deny that most cancers are serious, the idea that a diagnosis of cancer is a certain death warrant is now far from the truth. Most cancer deaths are avoidable through prevention or early diagnosis. Cancer covers about 200 different diseases, and although about one woman in three will develop a cancer at some time in her life, the most common forms are almost entirely preventable or treatable through early diagnosis. This Chapter looks at the cancers which are most common in women.

2 Bladder

1 The average age at diagnosis is 65 years. The good news is the cancer tends to spread slowly so the majority of tumours are still within the bladder at diagnosis. Even so early diagnosis improves the chances of survival.
2 A popular misperception is of the bladder as a simple bag to hold urine until a convenient convenience can be found. In fact it is a complex organ with delicate nervous control and intricate muscular layers. We tend to maltreat our bladders terribly expecting them to do their work without complaint. It is only

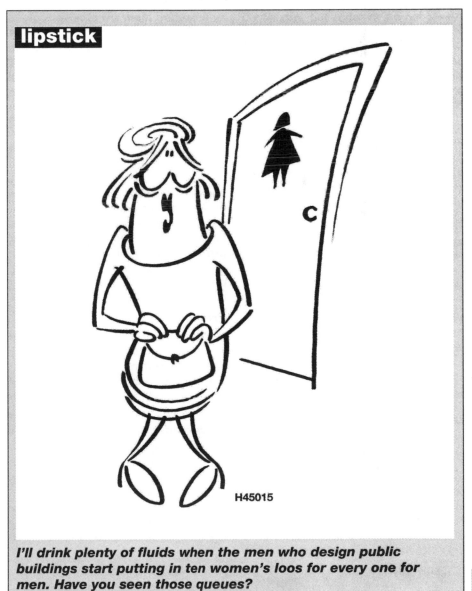

lipstick

H45015

I'll drink plenty of fluids when the men who design public buildings start putting in ten women's loos for every one for men. Have you seen those queues?

7

when things go wrong we realise just how important they are. Sitting low in the pelvis it sits immediately behind the pubis. It has three layers but it is the innermost layer in which cancer generally develops. A full bladder will hold around 350 ml (half a pint) of urine although some people can seem to store extra in their legs when stood at the bar. Voluntary control is amazingly good and pressures can rise inside the bladder to quite high levels before the point of no return is reached. There is no evidence that constantly holding on causes bladder cancer. Most cancers are caused by carcinogens carried either in the blood or in the urine. Obviously if they are in the urine they can be in contact with the inner layer of the bladder for quite some time, especially overnight. Drinking plenty of fluids helps flush out the carcinogens.

3 If the cancer is detected early and is present only in the innermost layer it can be cured by simple local treatment without opening the bladder (see *Diagnosis* below). Unfortunately, diagnosis at this stage is not common. After this the cancer will spread into the deeper layers and then eventually outside the bladder itself. Obviously this changes the outcome for successful treatment.

Symptoms

4 Pain is not a major feature of early bladder cancer even when passing blood or pus in the urine. Although these signs are also seen in less serious conditions, such as cystitis (bladder infection) they should always be taken seriously, especially when occurring for the first time in older women.

5 If left without early treatment more advanced bladder cancer may cause pain in the flanks (sides) or the loins, obstruction to the ureters, the tubes that carry urine down to the bladder from the kidneys, or bone pain from secondary cancer.

Causes

6 Although the causes of most bladder cancers remain uncertain some of them are known. These include:
• Cigarette smoking (the carcinogens are excreted in the urine). Heavy cigarette smoking is believed to be the cause in half the cases in women.
• Industrial chemicals such as aniline dyes, beta-naphthylamine and benzidine.

• Some chemicals encountered in rubber manufacture (tyre manufacture used to be a major risk). Artificial sweetener, once a suspect, is now known to be guiltless.
• Drugs such as phenacetin and cyclophosphamide (paradoxically used for treating cancer in other parts of the body).
• Possibly long-term bladder inflammation.
• Parasitic disease, especially schistosomiasis (a tropical parasite).
• Possibly the presence of bladder stones.
• Genetic. There is an increased risk if there is bladder cancer in the family.

Diagnosis

7 The symptoms will raise a doctor's suspicions and trigger further examination by specialists. Cystoscopy is examination of the inside of the urinary bladder by means of a fine telescope passed in through urethra. A general anaesthetic is available for most women.

8 Although no-one's idea of a good day out, this enables a distinction to be made between cancers (which are always dangerous) and bladder polyps (which are benign and simply harmless dangly bits within the bladder).

9 As some cells inevitably break off and travel in the urine these can be examined for the presence of cancer cells. Special X-rays using a radio-opaque dye that passes through the kidneys into the bladder may show any tumours inside the bladder.

Prevention

10 Bladder cancer is preventable and very treatable when caught early. Simply stopping smoking and taking proper precautions when using industrial chemicals will prevent most bladder cancers.

Treatment

11 When caught early with cancer confined to the inner surface of the bladder, a laser or burning with a hot wire (cautery) passed through a cystoscope can be curative. A washout of the bladder with anticancer drugs can also be highly effective but all need follow up to check for any resurfacing of cancer.

12 Surgery aims to eliminate all cancer, but this is not always possible. In about half of those people presenting with

signs of bladder cancer, the tumour is still in the early stages, is confined to the inner lining of the bladder and can readily be destroyed by direct surgery.

13 With spread through the wall of the bladder major surgery and radiotherapy will be needed. The whole bladder may have to be removed. As with all cancers early detection and prevention is vital.

2 Bowel

1 Although many people find it embarrassing to talk about symptoms of bowel problems, it is surprising how common they really are. There are lots of common conditions that could cause changes in the workings of the bowels, pain and bleeding from the bottom. In most cases, it won't be cancer.

2 Things women should know.
• Bowel cancer is the second most deadly cancer in the UK – only lung cancer kills more people. 35,600 people are diagnosed with the disease each year and over 45% will die as a result. That means that it claims the life of over 16,000 men and women in the UK each year. Bowel cancer is one of the most curable cancers if caught early. It's estimated that around 80% of cases could be treated successfully if caught at an early stage. Many people, often embarrassed to discuss their symptoms, delay seeking medical advice. It is vital to look out for possible symptoms and have them investigated (by a health professional such as a GP) if they persist.
• Basically divided into two parts, the bowel has 'small' and 'large' reflecting the width of the gut rather than its length. For some reason the small bowel is almost immune to cancer compared to the large bowel and rectum, the very last part of the digestive system.
• The large bowel is the question-mark shaped tube – about four feet long – which runs from the appendix, through the colon and down to the rectum and bowel cancer is cancer of any part of the colon or rectum that form most of the large intestine or bowel. If it is not treated, it will increase in size and may cause a blockage or can ulcerate leading to blood loss and anaemia.

• Most cancers start with wart-like growths known as polyps on the wall of the gut. Polyps are very common with age – one in ten people over 60 have them. However, most polyps do not turn into cancer. If potentially cancerous polyps can be found at an early stage, they can be removed painlessly without the need for an operation.

Symptoms

3 The most common symptoms are change of bowel habit and rectal bleeding. However, these are also common in people who don't have cancer, and around 20% of people experience bleeding from the bottom each year and over one third experience constipation or diarrhoea at some point in life.

4 There are some symptoms that need the attention of a doctor, especially if they last for longer than 6 weeks.

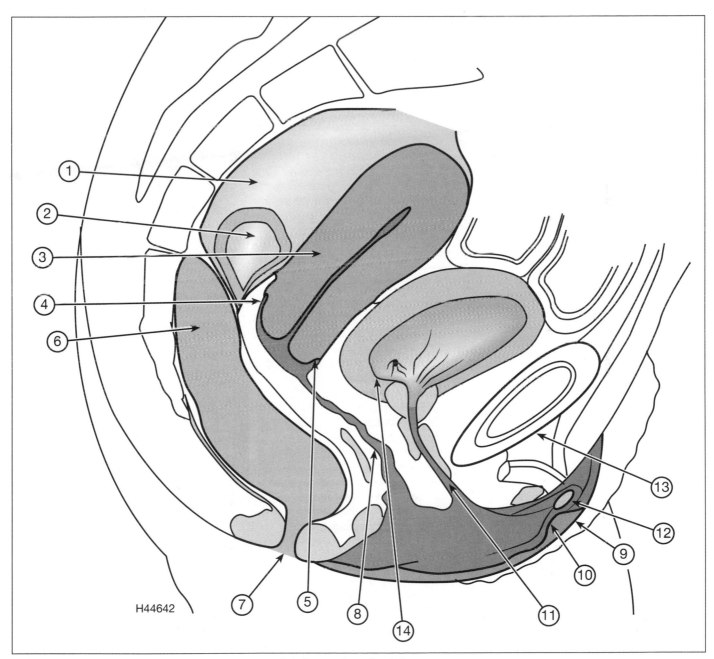

H44642

2.1 Lower female abdomen

1 Colon
2 Small intestine
3 Uterus
4 Posterior fornix
5 Anterior fornix
6 Rectum
7 Anus
8 Vagina
9 Labia majora
10 Labia minora
11 Urethra
12 Clitoris
13 Pubic bone
14 Bladder

7

- Change of bowel habit (especially important if you also have bleeding). Recent, persistent change of bowel habit to looser, more diarrhoea like motions, going to the toilet or trying to 'go' more often.
- Rectal bleeding that persists with no reason. For example, bleeding can be due to piles – but if so there may well be other symptoms such as straining with hard stools, a sore bottom, lumps and itching. In women over 60 piles could be hiding more serious symptoms, so it is especially important to get this investigated.
- Unexplained anaemia (see *Anaemia*).
- Lumps in the abdomen (tummy) especially when recognised by a GP.
- Persistent, severe abdominal pain which has come on recently for the first time (especially in older people but see *Abdominal pain*).

Causes

5 While bowel cancer can in some cases be put down to genetics, family history doesn't necessarily mean that a family member is going to get it. In general, the closer the relative (eg, brother, sister, mother, father, child) and the younger they were diagnosed, the more is the need to get it checked out.

6 The following is a guide to the action needed depending on family history:
- One close relative under 45 affected: It's worth talking to a GP about screening in the area. It is usually recommended 10 years before the age at which a relative developed the disease.
- Two or more close relatives from the same side of the family: The younger those relatives, the more need for discussing tests and screening with a GP.
- Less strong family history (such as a grandparent who died in their 70s) probably not at an increased risk, however any symptoms need a doctor's attention.
- Diet and lifestyle.

7 In many cases bowel cancer occurs without any obvious cause but experts

also suggest that a diet high in red meat and low in fibre, fruit and vegetables can increase the risk of bowel cancer. Obesity, high alcohol consumption and lack of physical exercise may increase the risk

Your risk increases if there is bowel cancer in the family but diet and smoking are among the main culprits.

Other causes

- Piles or haemorrhoids: Soft swellings, a bit like spongy varicose veins, which usually have other symptoms such as pain and itching. Bright red bleeding found on the toilet paper or sudden large amounts of blood are almost always caused by piles. Pharmacists will be able to recommend a fast and effective over-the-counter treatment (see *Piles*).
- Polyps: Warty-like growths on the bowel lining, which can sometimes cause bleeding. These can be removed painlessly without the need for an operation using a flexible telescope. There is some evidence however that they can lead on to bowel cancer so it is important to get them checked out.
- Fissures: A split or tear in the lining of the gut, sometimes caused by constipation and passing large hard stools. Fissures can be treated with creams available from the pharmacist but surgery may be required.
- Crohn's disease: Painful inflammation of the gut, which may increase the risk of bowel cancer so regular checks are important.
- Ulcerative colitis: Inflammation of the bowel which can cause bleeding and mucus. This condition may also be linked with a greater risk from bowel cancer.

8 Some things we do know increase your risk but the definite cause is still a mystery.
- A junk food diet high in fats and sugars and low in fibre.
- Bowel cancer in the close family.
- Lack of activity.
- Being overweight.
- Smoking tobacco.
- Having a bowel condition called polyps or adenomatous polyposis significantly increases your risk, even if in

another member of your family. Trying to pronounce it can be pretty stressful too.

Prevention

9 The good news is you can reduce your risk even if it is in the family.
- Check out your diet. Reduce the amount of fat and sugars and boost fruit and vegetables.
- Regular physical activity and keeping your weight under control.
- Any family history which increases your risk should be discussed with your doctor who may advise more frequent tests.
- Quit the weed.

Early detection gives best protection, so know your bum chum.

10 A high fibre diet is particularly recognised for reducing the risk of constipation, irritable bowel syndrome and bowel cancer. Fibre is indigestible plant material such as cellulose, lignin and pectin which is found in fruits, vegetables, grains and beans. There are two types of fibre – soluble and insoluble. Fibre provides bulk to food, helps it pass easily through the gut and also retains water.

11 Best evidence is that eating a minimum of 18g of fibre each day gives significant protection – yet most of people probably eat much less (around 10-12g). A banana contains 1.8g as does 1 slice of wholemeal toast.

12 Good ideas:
- Replacing lower fibre foods with high fibre foods, eg, whole grain breads and cereals.
- Eating vegetables and raw fruit whenever possible.
- Steaming or stir-frying vegetables has the edge over boiling, which can cause up to one half of the fibre to be lost in the water.
- Replacing fruit or vegetable juice with the whole fruit – fruit skin and membranes are a particularly good source of fibre.

Diagnosis

13 The GP may perform a Faecal Occult Blood test (looking for blood in the

It is not caused by sitting on hot radiators, eating vindaloo or even using newspaper for bog roll.

stools) and a DRE (digital rectal examination). Following these initial tests, if bowel cancer is suspected, patients will be referred for further tests.

• People with higher risk symptoms should be referred within two weeks for investigation. Most people with these symptoms do not have cancer but it should be ruled out by special tests.

• Most people will be sent to diagnostic clinics run by specialist nurses and doctors.

14 Specialist diagnostic investigations include:

• Flexible sigmoidoscopy: a thin flexible tube with a camera light on the end which can look inside the first 60 cm of the bowel.

• Colonoscopy: a long flexible tube to look inside the whole bowel. Laxatives are taken beforehand and no food is taken the day before to empty the bowel. The investigation is usually carried out under sedation.

• Barium enema: a special X-ray examination. The enema, a mixture of barium (a thick white liquid which shows up on X-ray) and air is passed through the back passage through a tube. Any abnormal areas show up black against the white liquid.

Coping and living with diagnosis

15 After initial diagnosis, you will discuss the options open to you with your specialist who will put together a treatment plan (depending on the type and size of the cancer, what stage the cancer is at and your personal health and age) including:

• When and where treatment will take place.

• What drugs will be available.

• Who will be treating you.

Surgery

16 During the operation a the piece of bowel that contains the cancer is removed and the two open ends are joined together. The lymph nodes near the bowel may also be removed because this is the first place to which the cancer may spread. Surgery can either be used alone or in combination with radiotherapy and chemotherapy.

Chemotherapy

17 This treatment uses anti-cancer drugs to destroy the cancer cells and is often given after surgery to reduce the

chances of the cancer coming back. It is also given when the cancer is advanced and has spread to other parts of the body.

18 Chemotherapy drugs cause different side-effects in different people. Some people may experience few side-effects and even those who do will only have these temporarily during treatment. Some of the common side-effects are tiredness, hair loss, mouth ulcers and nausea.

19 Chemotherapy is sometimes given with radiotherapy before surgery.

Radiotherapy

20 This treatment is usually used only to treat cancer of the rectum and can be given before or after surgery. Radiotherapy may also be given as a palliative treatment to relieve symptoms of the disease, eg, to reduce pain.

Colostomy bag

21 Most people diagnosed with bowel cancer do not need a colostomy bag – also called a stoma. Some people may need a temporary stoma but this can often be reversed after a few months. Although people need to time to adjust to having a stoma, life can carry on normal. Contact the British Colostomy Association for more information.

Chances of cancer returning

22 Following successful treatment, regular check-ups every few months are required to make sure that the cancer has not returned or spread.

23 If the bowel cancer was diagnosed and treated early there is a very good chance that it will not recur after treatment and even if the cancer does recur it can be treated with a combination of further surgery, chemotherapy or radiotherapy.

24 Five years with no return of the cancer is considered a cure.

Living with bowel cancer

25 There are many national and local charities, patient support groups and help lines which could offer you information, help and emotional support. See *Further information* for details.

Further information

26 If you would like to know more, look at the contacts section at the back of this book, or contact:

British Colostomy Association
Support, reassurance and practical information for people with a colostomy.
Helpline: 0800 328 4257
Tel: 0118 939 1537
Fax: 0118 923 9184
sue@bcass.org.uk
www.bcass.org.uk

National Association for Colitis and Crohn's Disease (NACC)
Tel: 0845 130 223
NACC in-Contact Support Line: 0845 130 3344
nacc@nacc.org.uk
www.nacc.org.uk

Digestive Disorders Foundation
Tel: 020 7486 0341
ddf@digestivedisorders.org.uk
www.digestivedisorders.org.uk

Ileostomy and Internal Pouch Support Group
Tel: 0800 018 4724
ia@ileostomypouch.demon.co.uk
www.ileostomypouch.demon.co.uk

3 Breasts

1 Breast cancer affects one in 50 women in the UK. Men can also have breast cancer, but it is relatively rare with around 150 cases each year. By way of contrast it is the most common type of cancer to affect women and, worldwide causes a million new cases every year. It is:

• Twice as common as cancer of the large intestine.

• Three times as common as lung and womb lining cancer.

• Four times as common as cancer of the ovary.

• Each year more than 14,000 women in Britain die from breast cancer (around 10,000 men die from prostate cancer).

• It is the single commonest cause of death among women in the age-range 40 to 50.

• The percentage of deaths among women resulting from breast cancer rises steadily to the age of 45 and then declines.

2 Yet, despite all this there is an overblown fear. When asked most women thought breast cancer was a greater risk of death than heart disease. In fact the reverse is true.

3 It helps to know how the breast works. The human breast consists of 15 to 20 lobes each with its terminal duct along which the milk passes during breast feeding. These ducts are lined with cells called epithelial cells which sit on a transparent membrane called the epithelial basement membrane. Breast cancers are cancers of these epithelial cells.

4 These lobes are held together by fibrous tissue and a variable amount of fatty tissue that is largely responsible for the differences in the size of different breasts. During pregnancy the overall size of the breast increases. The ducts from the different lobes converge on the nipple and each passes independently through the nipple to the exterior.

5 When a cancer starts in the ductal epithelial cells it is, for some time, confined to that layer. Such a cancer is called carcinoma in situ (CIN) and it has not yet spread. Only once it has spread it is said to be an invasive cancer.

6 By examining a sample of the cancer tissue by microscope it is possible to grade it in terms of malignancy. Breast cancers differ in the speed with which they spread locally and remotely. These differences are called degrees of malignancy.

7 The greater the irregularity and the greater the proportion that are dividing, the higher the malignancy. In this way, experts can divide breast cancers into three grades, Grades I, II and III. Grade I cancers are the least malignant; grade III are the most malignant. Predictions of survival can be made based on this fundamental difference in the way the tumour is behaving.

8 On average, five years after diagnosis:
*   Over 90 per cent of the women with Grade I tumours have survived.
*   With Grade II tumours about 70 per cent have survived.
*   With Grade III tumours just under 50 per cent have survived.

9 Fourteen years after diagnosis:
*   Over 80 per cent of women with Grade I tumours have survived.
*   Around 48 per cent of those with Grade II tumours have survived.
*   Around 42 per cent of those with Grade III tumours have survived.

10 The size of the cancer is also one of the most important factors.

*   Tumours less than 2 cm across at the time of diagnosis and treatment will show 60 per cent of women free of recurrences five years later.
*   Tumours 2-5 cm across will show about 40 per cent of the women free of recurrence at five years.
*   Tumours more than 5 cm across will show about 20 per cent of women free of recurrence at five years.

11 It is not quite so simple as this, in addition to the grades of malignancy, breast cancers are assessed in terms of the stage they have reached at the time of diagnosis. This is a complex process taking into account such factors as whether the cancer is invasive; the size of the tumour; whether or not it has spread to the lymph nodes; whether or not blood and liver function tests, chest X-rays and scans suggest remote spread (metastases).

12 Early diagnosis is vital. Women who delay for more than three months after finding a lump, subsequently proved to be cancer, have a substantially lower survival rate than those who report the problem within three months.

Symptoms

13 Unfortunately like many cancers, breast cancers produce few warning signs and rarely cause pain, one of the most important reasons for people to see their doctor. There may, sometimes, be a vague discomfort, but, commonly, the only sign is the finding of a slowly growing lump. There are, however, other possible signs and these should be known and looked for. They are:
*   A change in the outline, shape or size of the breast.
*   A new isolated lump.
*   Change of the normal breast outline by skin dimpling.
*   In-drawing, or alteration in direction, of the nipple.
*   Persistent discharge or bleeding from the nipple.
*   Distortion of the area around the nipple (areola).
*   Orange-skin appearance of the breast skin.
*   Alteration in the position or hang of the breast compared to the other side.
*   Rubbery, firm, easily felt glands (lymph nodes) in the armpit.

Causes

14 The great variation in breast cancer rates from country to country is a great reason for optimism. The death rate from breast cancer in India, for instance, is only about 20 per 100,000. In Singapore Chinese it is about 30 per 100,000; in Brazil 40 per 100,000; in Finland 50 per 100,000; in Scotland 62 per 100,000; in Iceland 70 per 100,000 and in USA nearly 90 per 100,000. Moving from a low rate country to a high rate country exposes women, and their offspring, to the higher rate. Within two generations the rate of breast cancer in immigrants reaches the standard rate in the country they are now living in. This finding suggests that environmental factors are more important than genetic factors in producing breast cancer. It means that potentially we can do a lot more about it.

15 There are factors known to increase the risk of breast cancer. These include:
*   Early start to menstruation, before age 11 (three times the risk).
*   Late menopause, after 54 (twice the risk).
*   Having a first child late (three times the risk).
*   Exposure to radiation (three times the risk).
*   Being overweight after the menopause (twice the risk).
*   Cancer in the other breast (more than four times the risk).
*   Previous non-cancer disease of breast (four times the risk).
*   Exposure to atomic (ionising) radiation (three times the risk).
*   Breast cancer in mother, sister or daughter diagnosed under the age of 50 (twice the risk).

16 There is also a genetic risk, a family history of breast cancer is an important factor. Families which, in three generations, have four or more relatives with either breast or ovarian cancer and one alive relative with one of these cancers, should be considered for gene testing. About 10 per cent of breast cancers have a genetic basis. Women with a strong family history of breast cancer of early onset, but who reach the age of 65 without developing breast cancer have probably not inherited the gene mutations that cause breast cancer.

17 Where you both live can be a big factor. Living in a developed country significantly increases the risk of breast cancer. Western high-fat diet may be an important reason for the higher incidence. Also, women tend to have babies later in life.

18 Women living on a diet high in fruit and vegetables and low in dairy fats and dairy products are less likely to get breast cancer than women whose diets are high in dairy fats. Research suggests that diets high in total fats, and diets high in saturated fat, increase the risk of breast cancer. Diets high in olive oil may reduce the risk.

19 Oral contraceptives very slightly increases the risk, as does hormone replacement therapy (HRT) although recent evidence suggests that this risk increases with prolonged use of hormone replacement. Consult a doctor.

Diagnosis and screening

20 Mammographs (breast X-rays) are important but whoever invented this damn machine certainly didn't have breasts!

21 Mammography cannot give a definitive diagnosis, this is done by microscopic examination of a biopsy (sample). Tissue may be obtained by sucking out some cells through a fine needle inserted into the lump under a local anaesthetic.

22 Mammography is the only screening test available for breast cancer which has been shown in trials to reduce breast cancer deaths. Experts now believe that mammography, if properly done, can reduce the mortality from breast cancer by up to 40 per cent in women aged 50 to 70 who attend for screening. The object is to detect cancer at the earliest possible stage before it has spread out of the breast. Women aged 50-70 are invited every three years. Older women can still be screened on request.

23 If something suspicious is seen at basic screening, women are recalled for assessment of the abnormality. This can include a clinical examination of the breast, an ultrasound scan and possibly taking a few cells out of the breast in clinic to examine under a microscope. Seven out of eight women called back do not have cancer.

24 For every thousand women screened, about 6 will be found to have invasive breast cancer and one will be found to have "carcinoma in situ", this is an early abnormality which is still confined to the ducts of the breast and has not yet started to invade surrounding breast tissue.

Prevention

25 Breast awareness is the name of the game for survival but it doesn't actually prevent breast cancer. Addressing risk factors is the only real prevention although research suggests that the drug tamoxifen may reduce the risk of breast cancer. It was noted that in trials of tamoxifen as an additional measure in the treatment of actual breast cancer, the number of cancers occurring in the other breast was fewer than would normally be expected. This is still highly speculative.

Treatment

26 Past treatments of breast cancer were associated with dreadful disfiguration with equally dreadfully poor results. Conventional treatment of breast cancer has been by radical mastectomy, an aggressive surgical removal of all breast tissue and connected lymph nodes together with the removal of the underlying chest muscles (pectorals). Evidence based surgery has shown that less mutilating operations and various combinations of radiotherapy, anti-cancer chemotherapy, hormone treatment and immune system boosting can produce far better results.

27 In recent years there has been a trend towards even less mutilating operations and it is now common to employ a simple removal of the mass (lumpectomy) followed by a course of radiotherapy using linear accelerators or a cobalt 60 source. The study of the results of such methods shows that they can be as successful as radical mastectomy and that cancerous nodes can be treated just as effectively by radiation as by operation.

Man & Woman

28 Recognising the fear breast cancer can produce in a woman is the first part of addressing the problem together. This is a cancer which often strikes women in their relative youth and in a bodily place of obvious femininity. Supporting her through the process of diagnosis, treatment and recovery especially after mastectomy makes all the difference.

29 Men like women's breasts because they look and feel nice, but for women they can be the foundation of their femininity. Growing them tells us we've grown up, having them makes us feel sexy and with them we give and receive pleasure and feed our children. The thought of losing one or both can fill us with terror and disgust, which is why many of us shy away from the very thought of breast cancer and avoid tests. Support your woman in having tests.

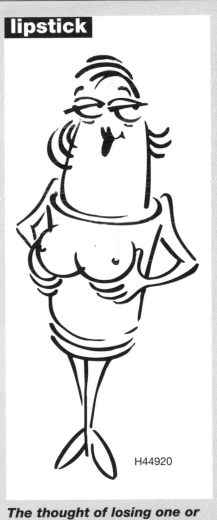

lipstick

H44920

The thought of losing one or both breasts can fill women with terror and disgust, which is why many shy away from the very thought of breast cancer and avoid tests

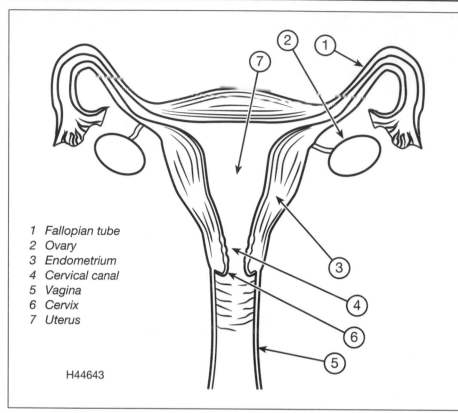

1 Fallopian tube
2 Ovary
3 Endometrium
4 Cervical canal
5 Vagina
6 Cervix
7 Uterus

H44643

4.1 Female reproductive organs

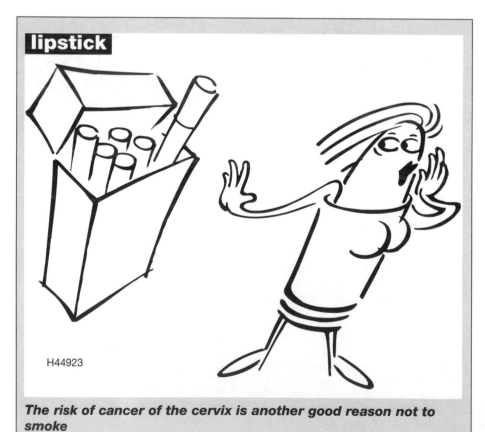

lipstick

H44923

The risk of cancer of the cervix is another good reason not to smoke

4   Cervix

1   Cancer of the neck of the womb (cervix) is unfortunately not rare and is second only to cancer of the breast with around 2000 women dying each year in Britain and the number of women developing the cancer is on the increase. As there is an effective screening process these deaths are particularly tragic as most of them are preventable with early detection and treatment. It is a thankfully slow-growing cancer and is preceded for many years by a recognizable and easily diagnosable pre-invasive (malignant) condition, known as carcinoma in situ (CIN). Half of all cancers of the female reproductive system are in the cervix.

Symptoms

2   Unfortunately, like others, cancer of the cervix often causes no symptoms until it has spread and may have no symptoms at all before reaching an incurable stage.

3   Perhaps the most significant symptom is bleeding between periods, following sexual intercourse or after the menopause, all of which need to be reported to the doctor. Pain and general upset are rare until a late stage is reached. These are the most important reasons for regular cervical screening.

Causes

4   The following increase the risk of developing cervical cancer:
•   Genital warts.
•   Multiple sexual partners.
•   Sex with a partner who has genital warts.
•   Smoking.
•   Pregnancy at an early age.
•   Having three or more pregnancies.
•   Virus infection may also play a part, in particular two viruses may be linked, the human papilloma (wart) virus and the herpes simplex (genital herpes) virus.

5   The risk of cancer of the cervix is another good reason not to smoke.

Diagnosis

6   This is made by direct examination, and by taking a biopsy for microscopic examination.

Screening

7 All women who have ever had sex with a man should have regular cervical screening (the 'Pap' or 'smear' test). Cervical screening aims to prevent cancer developing by finding and treating cervical abnormalities before they can develop into cancer.

8 Women should have their first test at 25 and then every three years after that until the age of 50, when they only require them every 5 years until the age of 64. After that, if all recent tests have been clear, then a woman can safely stop going for screening. The "smear test" is currently being replaced by newer liquid based tests which have a much lower "inadequate" rate and which labs can process more quickly giving results to women in a shorter time period

9 If a test is not found to be entirely normal, a woman might be recommended to have another test after a short interval or might be referred for colposcopy. This is an examination of the cervix in clinic by a gynaecologist who will then be able to recommend any further action, or possibly treat the abnormality there and then.

Complications

10 Although early diagnosis and treatment is almost always successful, spread of the cancer to other organs in the pelvis and further afield is common, although modern treatments are extending life expectancy for many women.

Treatment

11 Early diagnosis and treatment is vital as established cancer is difficult to treat successfully and the jury is still out over which is the best form of treatment, surgery or radiotherapy. Radiotherapy is widely used and this is usually provided by means of sealed containers of radioactive caesium or radium that are placed inside the vagina and womb.

12 Success depends in the main on the extent of spread at the time of diagnosis.

Early cancer, confined to the cervix, offers an excellent prognosis, with a cure rate of over 85 per cent. But if there has been spread to the vagina and surrounding tissues, the cure rate drops to about 50 per cent.

13 Sadly, a more extensive spread to the organs of the pelvis, and particularly remote spread to other parts of the body, has a very poor outlook. In only about ten per cent of such cases is the patient still alive five years later.

5 Larynx

1 Well known as the Adam's Apple, the larynx is the box-like structure at the top of the windpipe. Partly composed of gristle (cartilage) it has a prominent front part, especially in men. It has two important jobs, making noise with the vocal cords for the mouth and tongue to turn into speech and stopping food going down 'the wrong way'. Trying to do both at the same time is one of the tricky bits which can go wrong, especially after a few pints of lager and faced with large chunks of poorly chewed steak. It has sensitive nerves which triggering coughing when spaghetti Bolognese is boldly going where air should only go.

2 Although relatively rare, cancer of the larynx occurs most often in smokers and heavy drinkers. If the cancer is confined to the vocal cords it causes obvious voice changes and is likely to be diagnosed early. In addition, spread from the vocal cords to other parts is thankfully slow. In this case the outlook is favourable. Unfortunately, cancer elsewhere in the larynx is likely to be well advanced before symptoms of breathing or swallowing difficulty arise so the prospects of a cure is not so good.

Symptoms

3 An obvious symptom of cancer of the larynx is a change in the voice. This is not the usual sore throat of an infection or after speaking for long periods. Singers and actors know this feeling well. With cancer there is a permanent hoarseness. With a longer standing cancer there can be difficulty in breathing and swallowing.

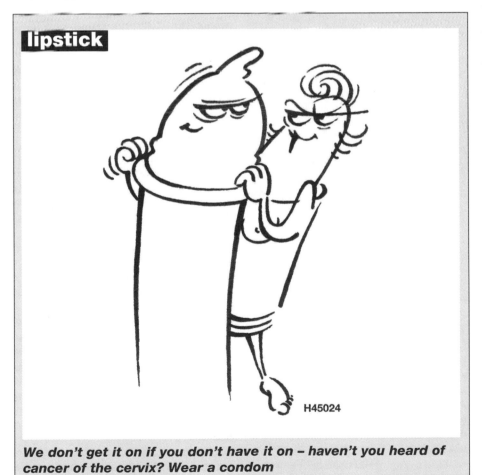

lipstick

We don't get it on if you don't have it on – haven't you heard of cancer of the cervix? Wear a condom

H45024

7

Causes

4 Tobacco smoking is the single greatest cause but others include alcohol abuse and exposure to asbestos fibres. Obviously stopping smoking, drinking in moderation and using mixers rather than drinking neat spirits makes sense.

Diagnosis

5 Any marked change in the voice lasting more than a couple of weeks should be investigated by an expert without delay. It is possible to look at the inside of the larynx using an instrument called a fibre optic laryngoscope and any cancer present is generally readily visible.

Prevention

6 Laryngeal cancer is almost totally preventable by stopping smoking, drinking in moderation and avoiding neat spirits.

Treatment

7 Early diagnosis is essential as small cancers of the vocal cords can often be cured by local treatment with lasers or, more often, with radiotherapy. Larger cancers that have spread to involve the cartilage of the larynx usually require partial or total removal of the larynx (laryngectomy). Obviously this means the vocal cords are no longer there to vibrate and produce the sounds acted on by the mouth for speech. This is where the latest technology steps in with electromechanical devices that mimic their function. Speech therapists can give invaluable support and advice.

6 Lungs

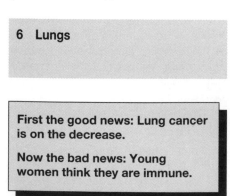

First the good news: Lung cancer is on the decrease.

Now the bad news: Young women think they are immune.

1 Most people think of the lungs as two plastic bags or balloons. Nothing could be further from the truth. Lungs are complex structures with more similarity

You do not get permanently fat when you stop smoking but you do enjoy your food more.

to sponges than balloons. The main pipe (bronchus) connects both lungs to the airway in the throat. It splits lower in the chest branching increasingly until tiny blind ending pockets are reached. These are the alveoli and oxygen is exchanged for carbon dioxide across the thin membranes. Cancer can arise in the fine tubes but mainly in the larger tubes, the bronchi.

2 The correct medical term for lung cancer is bronchial carcinoma, a cancer of the large tubes of the lung. The lining cells of the air tubes in healthy lungs are tall (columnar) and the surfaces nearest the inside of the tube are covered with fine hairs (cilia) which move together. Imagine a wind blowing across a field of ripe corn. The movement of the cilia acts to carry dust and smoke particles and other foreign material upwards and away from the deeper parts of the lungs. This is essential to keep the lungs clear of debris and potentially harmful particles.

3 Smoking cigarettes damages the lung's ability to do their jobs. First, the cilia disappear, then the number of cells increases and, finally, the cells become flattened, so that the columnar lining is replaced by an abnormal, scaly layer. Some years later it may develop into bronchial carcinoma.

4 Lung cancer is uncommon before the age of 40. Only about 1 case in 100 is diagnosed in people younger than 40. The great majority of cases (85 per cent) occur in people over 60.

5 The outlook in lung cancer is not good. After diagnosis of the disease 20 per cent are alive a year later, and only 8 per cent, overall, survive for five years.

The Smoking Gun

• It's not difficult to work out what causes it. If you don't smoke the chances of getting lung cancer are very small.

• Start early, die early and the amount of tobacco smoked also shifts a person that bit closer to the great scrapyard in the sky.

• Filters and low tar protect? Far from it – they give a false sense of security (ever

watched a film of the hero going into a fume filled room with a wet hanky over his mouth?).

• Cut down then? Nah, doesn't work either. It gradually creeps back up. You both need to stop completely.

6 All over the UK women are getting the message but it often needs support to ensure success.

Symptoms

7 Lung cancer usually shows itself with a productive cough and there is often a little blood in the sputum. There may also be breathlessness. Pain in the chest is common, especially if the cancer has spread to the lung lining (pleura) or the chest wall.

8 Unfortunately the tumour may show no signs until late in its development.

9 Watch out for:
• A persistent cough.
• Coughing up blood stained phlegm (sputum).
• Shortness of breath.
• Chest discomfort.
• Repeated bouts of pneumonia or bronchitis.
• Loss of appetite.
• Loss of weight.

10 These don't necessarily mean there is cancer but they need a doctor's attention in case further tests are needed.

Causes

11 It is almost entirely due to cigarette smoking although passive smoking is another known cause. The rate of lung cancer in non-smokers rises significantly if they are regularly exposed to other people's cigarette smoke.

Diagnosis

12 Unfortunately diagnosis tends to be late in the day and can be fairly obvious from the symptoms described to a doctor. X-ray examination will often confirm the diagnosis although sometimes the diagnosis can only be made by examining the inside of the bronchi with a bronchoscope. If a tumour is seen, a sample (biopsy) is usually taken for examination. Cancer cells can sometimes be found in the sputum.

13 Treatment will depend on the type of cancer, how developed it is and general state of health. Surgery, radiotherapy

and chemotherapy may be used alone or together to treat cancer of the lung.
• Surgery: removal of part or all of the lung
• Radiotherapy: the use of radiation treatment to destroy cancer cells.
• Chemotherapy: the use of drugs that kill cancer cells.

Prevention

14 Nobody is trying to kid you that any of these treatments guarantee a cure but early detection of the cancer can make all the difference.
15 Better still, reduce the risk of getting it in the first place by both stopping smoking.

How to quit the weed

• Nicotine patches and other ways of helping to stop can be obtained through the GP. These can be very successful in easing the craving for nicotine.
• Get in touch with self-help groups or organisations which supply information.
• If she can't do it for herself, ask her to do it for you or the kids.

Quit plan

• Set a day and date to stop. Tell all the friends and relatives, they will give support.
• Like deep sea diving, always have a buddy. Get someone to give up with her. It will reinforce each other's willpower.
• Clear the house of any packets, papers or matches.
• One day at a time is better than leaving it open-ended.
• Map out progress on a chart or calendar.
• Encourage her to keep the money saved in a separate container.
• Offer carrots to chew on. It will it help her to do something with her mouth and hands.
• Ask your friends not to smoke around you both. People accept this far more readily than they used to do.

I smoke because it feels like a treat – time out and something just for me. You want to help me give up? Let's find something else that gives me that feeling. Give me a foot rub, run me a bath, buy me a CD and let me listen for 10 minutes.

7 Malignant melanoma

1 This nasty skin cancer is on the big increase. Prevention and, failing that, early diagnosis are vital. Only mad dogs and Englishmen go out in the midday sun, but English women are catching up quick. Being aware of the potential problem and having an insight into what is going on is important.
2 There are two main layers in the skin:
• The inner layer called the dermis, and the outer layer, the epidermis. At the base of the epidermis is a single layer of active cells called the basal layer. This layer buds off new cells that are then pushed towards the surface, becoming flatter and harder as they move outwards eventually dying forming an imperious covering to the more vulnerable skin below. This is the 'wear and tear' layer of the skin, and the cells on the surface are cast off.
• The pigmented cells in the basal layer are called melanocytes. These cells contain a brown colouring matter (pigment) called melanin giving the skin its darker colour. A melanoma is a tumour that starts in one of these cells.
3 Although still comparatively rare, melanoma will affect around 5 to 10 per 100,000 of the white population per year. The incidence in people under 20 is low (about two per cent). White people are at 10 to 20 times greater risk than are black and dark-skinned peoples.
4 The last 25 years saw the number of cases of malignant melanoma increase more rapidly than that of any other tumour. The increases are greatest in adolescents and young adults. By far the most likely explanation of this is the increasing affluence in the Western world, and the suntan culture, that have led to a marked increase in skin exposure to sunlight, holes in the ozone layer coming a close second. Cancer is unfortunately relatively common but only one cancer in 100 is a malignant melanoma. Even so, this has doubled every ten years for the past 40 years.
5 Nearly everyone has pigmented moles and about half of malignant

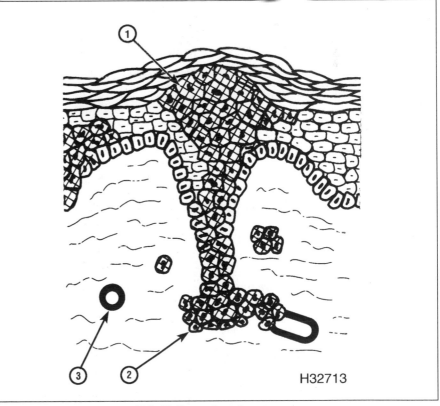

7.1 Malignant melanoma
1 Cancer cells in epidermis   2 Cancer cells spreading into dermis   3 Blood vessel

melanomas arise from pre-existing moles, but only one in a million becomes malignant. Better still, moles with lots of hairs growing through them hardly ever turn into malignant melanomas. Delay is the killer, once suspicious of changes in a coloured skin mole, seek an expert opinion as soon as possible.

Symptoms

6 In white people, malignant melanomas occur most often on the upper part of the back. In women, it is also equally common on the legs between the ankle and the knee. In black people, melanomas a very rare but when they do occur they are usually on the palms, soles and behind the finger and toe nails.

7 The signs of malignant change in a mole are very important to know. They are:

• Changes in shape, especially an increasingly irregular, rough outline.
• Changes in size, often losing any circular shape.
• Changes in texture feeling raised above the skin.
• Changes in colour, especially sudden darkening and the development of colour irregularities appearing as different shades of brown, grey, pink, red or blue.
• Sudden itching or pain not previously present.
• Smaller moles forming around the original one.
• A light or dark halo or ring forming around the mole.

8 Any one of these changes needs the attention of a doctor.

Causes

9 Skin most exposed to the sun are the most common at risk areas but it can occur anywhere on the skin. There is a definite link between sunbathing and the incidence of malignant melanomas. Probably the most dangerous type of sunbathing is a short, sharp period of intense exposure, either in a single day or over a short period such as a holiday.

10 Some white people are more likely to get melanomas than others. People with freckles, those with 20 or more birthmarks, and those who have had 3 or more severe sunburns, are at least 200 times more likely to get a melanoma than those with none of these features.

Diagnosis

11 Simply looking at a suspect mole is not enough, there is only one way to make a positive and sure diagnosis of a malignant melanoma, a total biopsy of the suspected tumour where the whole suspected tumour is removed and then examined. Checking the margins of the biopsy gives a good idea Margins of normal skin should be left all round. In this way the whole specimen is available for examination.

Prevention

12 Cover up. Fair skin along with inappropriate exposure to the sun with burning are the big dangers. Sunbeds are now highly suspect.

13 T-shirts or other protective clothing should be worn during swimming but watch out for thin material which can still let dangerous amounts of sun radiation through. Effective sunscreen creams should be used, forget about the lower factor stuff they only give a false sense of security. Stay indoors during the midday period when the sun's rays pass through the thinnest atmospheric distance and are thus most intense. Use high factor sunscreen creams but don't rely on them to protect entirely. It is better to avoid the direct rays of the sun or wear a hat and clothing.

Treatment

14 Biopsy is often the treatment as a wide area of normal-seeming tissue is also removed around the mole. Early diagnosis gives a very good chance of survival, in cases of treated melanomas with a thickness of 1 mm or less, the survival rate is 90 per cent.

8 Ovaries

1 For reasons we are still not sure of, cancer of the ovary is commoner in women who have never had children than in those who have. A similar pattern with breast cancer which early pregnancy seems to protect. It may occur at any age but is most usual between 50 and 80. Before age 30, the incidence is less than 1 per 50,000; after 55 it is about 1 per 2000 women. The greatest risk is for women in their 70s.

2 Mystery still revolves around the fact that oral contraceptives reduces the risk to a quarter. The condition tends slightly to run in families and a woman with one close relative with the disease has twice the general risk of getting it.

Symptoms

3 Like other cancers, ovarian cancer tends to be 'silent' until it has grown and spread, either putting pressure on and invading the womb (uterus) or spreading widely within the pelvis and abdomen. About two-thirds of women with the disease already have it spread beyond the pelvis when they see their doctor for diagnosis.

When there are symptoms they tend to be abdominal pain and discomfort, weight loss and urinary symptoms.

Causes

4 There may well be a genetic origin and the same genes as are implicated in genetic breast cancer but in most cases the cause is still unknown. The

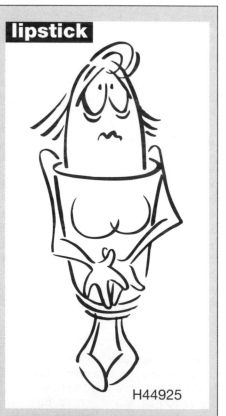

lipstick

H44925

I know she may think it's a drag, but if your woman has that 'dragging' feeling, help her get it checked out

relationship between breast cancer and HRT may well be a cause for investigation with an possible link with ovarian cancer as well. Research is checking this out.

Diagnosis

5 Endoscopic visualisation (laparoscopy) using a flexible telescope inserted through a small cut in the abdomen under general anaesthetic is the best way of confirming any presence of cancer although ultrasound can be used for early diagnosis. Early diagnosis is becoming increasingly possible through advances in screening for ovarian cancer with blood tests for specific markers of the cancer.

Treatment

6 Surgery is the only realistic treatment at present with the womb and both ovaries removed, as the second ovary often also contains tumour. Ovarian cancer often responds very well to anti-cancer chemotherapy but early diagnosis and treatment is essential for a success.

9 Pituitary

1 Often described as the 'body's orchestral conductor' the pituitary is a complex gland sitting at the base of the brain. It produces a number of hormones which collectively determine to a large extent the way the body functions. Cancer of this important part of the brain is fortunately rare and is increasingly more successful to treat. The effect of the tumour will depend on whether or not it produces hormones which act on distant parts of the body. Most cancers are non malignant so spread from the gland is not a problem. Even so, the hormones they produce or the pressure from the size of the tumour can cause their own serious problems.

Symptoms

2 These will depend on the type of tumour, the hormone it is producing or preventing and any pressure on surrounding tissues.

• Infertility can result from excess or lack of production of hormones.
• Excess stimulation of the adrenal glands near the kidney can produce a condition called 'Cushing's Syndrome' with characteristic 'moon face' appearance and high blood pressure.
• Visual disturbances can occur from pressure on the optic nerves which run very close to the pituitary.
• Lack of stimulation of the thyroid gland in the neck can lead to lethargy, thick skin and weight gain.

Diagnosis

3 The warning signs for the doctor will come from what is described as happening. These can take place over a prolonged period of time so the penny doesn't always drop immediately. Blood tests for abnormally low or high levels of hormones can provide invaluable clues but MRI or CT scans of the brain can often show the tumour. Although these tumours tend to be slow growing early diagnosis makes successful treatment all the more likely.

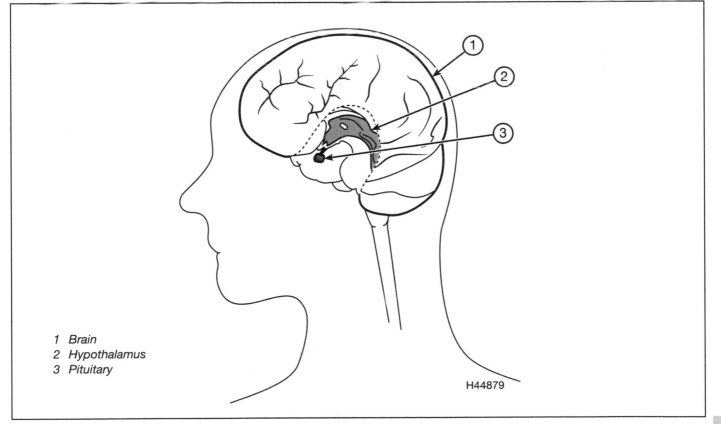

1 Brain
2 Hypothalamus
3 Pituitary

H44879

9.1 The pituitary gland

Treatment

4 A great deal depends on the type of tumour. Chemotherapy, radiotherapy and surgery are used often together and this may require hormone replacement on a regular basis to make up for the loss of tissue that normally produce the essential hormones.

10 Skin

See that big round yellow thing hanging in the sky? It causes more cancer in the UK than anything else you can shake a pair of sunglasses at.

Don't be a mad dog, get out of the midday sun!

Sunscreens and smokescreens

1 People get confused over sunscreens and can damage their skin through a false sense of security, remember:

• The higher the Sun Protection Factor (SPF) number, the greater the protection provided. A SPF above 15 gives high protection.

Not a lot of people know this

- *Skin cancer is the most common cancer in the UK.*
- *The risk of growing an extra, unwanted, outside cancerous lump by the age of 74 is one in six.*
- *Even cloudy days can deliver 9/10ths of the dangerous UV rays.*
- *Some tops are so thin they let almost all the sun's UV radiation shine right through.*
- *Once the sunburn fades from this year's trip to Majorca it doesn't mean you're in the clear. Damage builds up under the skin to cause problems later in life.*
- *Virtually all the risk comes from the sun and sunbeds... So cover up and close up!*

Shades of the truth

- *Use high factor sun-screens (30+) . Slap loads on BEFORE heading into the sun and re-apply every 2 hours*
- *Cover up, always, and that means when working or holidaying at home too.*
- *Get ahead and get a hat, a big hat.*
- *Get out of the midday sun when possible or else look for a nice bit of shade to relax or work in.*
- *Get those shades on to protect the (next) best assets!*

All women, no matter what colour their skin, need to be sun smart but those with:

- *Pale or freckled skin that doesn't tan, or burns before it tans.*
- *Naturally red or fair hair and blue, green or grey eyes.*
- *A large number of moles (50 or more).*
- *Easily burnt skin, a history of sunburn or who have already had skin cancer.*

need to be extra careful even when working or playing outside.

• Wearing sunscreen does not mean that you can stay out in the sun longer than recommended – it offers some protection, but should be used with cover-up clothing.

• It is very important to apply sunscreen thickly and evenly. Most people get a lot less protection than they think because they do not put enough sunscreen on their skin.

• Those parts of the body that are not usually exposed to the sun will tend to burn more easily. But also take extra care of ears, neck, hands and feet.

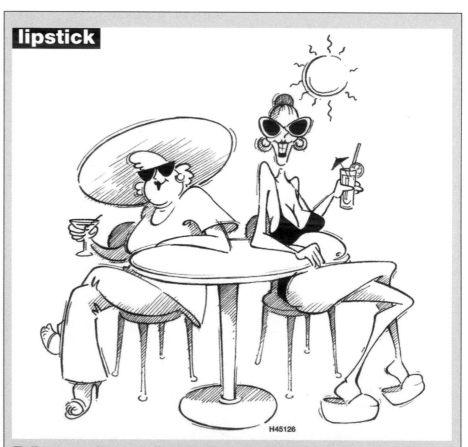

lipstick

H45126

Tell me you love my English Rose complexion. Keep drooling over suntans and that only makes me take risks

Sun Sense

2 The sun damages skin by its Ultraviolet Radiation (UV) and there are two types:

UVA

• Results in early ageing and skin cancer.

UVB

• Most harmful, causes burning and skin cancer.

3 Tanned skin is damaged skin. It's a sign that damaged skin is trying to protect itself from the sun's ultraviolet rays. Even when you have a suntan, you can still get sunburn.

4 There are two main types of skin cancer:

Non-Melanoma Skin Cancer

5 Most common form, often seen on the ear tips, nose, forehead and cheeks but is very curable.

6 Look out for:

• A new growth or sore that does not heal within four weeks.

• A spot or sore that continues to itch, hurt, crust, scab or bleed.

• Constant skin ulcers that are not explained by other causes.

Malignant Melanoma

7 See *Malignant melanoma*.

11 Thyroid

1 The thyroid gland sits in the throat just below the Adams Apple (larynx). It has the job of regulating the body's metabolism. Too much thyroxine – its secreted hormone – and the body works too fast with the heart beating too quickly. Too little and the body is sluggish with a slow heart rate. Cancer of the thyroid is more common in women and previous exposure to radiation may be part of the cause. It is rare, one in 100 of all cancers are of the thyroid. It is more common in people over 40 years old. The good news is that successful treatment for thyroid cancer is amongst the highest for any cancers.

Symptoms

2 These depend on the type of thyroid cancer as they can arise in different parts of the gland. The majority tend to spread outside of the gland itself. Symptoms include:

• A painless lump in the throat.

• Difficulty or pain on swallowing.

• Hoarse voice.

Causes

3 There are no known causes of thyroid cancer other than the possible effect of direct radiation. Therefore there is little to advise on prevention. Thankfully it is a rare cancer.

Diagnosis

4 Examination of the neck and blood tests by a GP will provide most clues to the diagnosis but ultrasound, MRI or CT scanning can give definitive diagnosis particularly after a biopsy (taking a small sample of thyroid tissue).

Treatment

5 Surgical removal of the entire gland will often make survival possible. This can be done along side radioactive iodine which will only affect the thyroid gland or the metastases. As a result thyroxine replacement, the normal hormone produced by the thyroid gland, will be needed. Around 95% of people will survive their cancer.

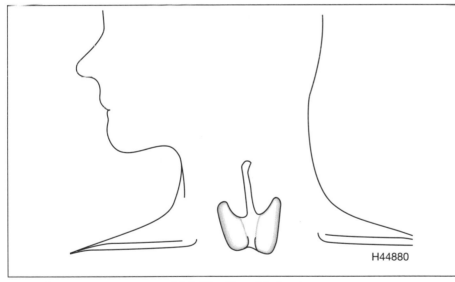

H44880

11.1 The thyroid gland

12 Obesity

See Chapter 2.

Reference

Contents

Contacts

Websites

There's a massive amount of material out there on the web but where do you start sorting through it? The information needs of a newly-diagnosed patient are different from those of someone who's had the disease for some time, the needs of a relative are different from those of a health professional.

So where do you begin to look for the information that you personally need? This section will help you to answer that question.

Search engine tips

The web is like an enormous library but although you're permitted to take out most of the books, there is no index system to help you find them. At best search engines trawl barely a third of the resources on the internet, often a lot less. So while your preferred search engine may be quick, its results are no better than those of an assistant with reasonable knowledge of a small corner of the library.

To get the best out of a search engine, try to be specific. Use the 'advanced search' option if available. This may allow you to select only UK sites or only those updated in, say, the last three months. This not necessarily because you are only interested in new information, but because you may well want to avoid dormant sites which are no longer being updated.

You aren't restricted to searching for individual words. You can use quotation marks to search for specific phrases. For example, to search for "breast cancer". Also use + (plus) and - (dash/minus) to narrow down your results; note that the plus or minus signs must have no space after them. For example: 'breast +cancer' will retrieve items that mention both breasts and cancer. The minus command might help if, for example, you wanted to find research by your doctor, the unfortunately named Dr Jekyll, but didn't want to be inundated with Robert Louis Stevenson references. You could try "Dr Jekyll" -"Mr Hyde"

A combination of the above can be very powerful indeed, enabling pinpoint searches. For example, "breast cancer" +"Dr Jekyll" +"Belchester Bugle" could help you to track down that article your friend reckoned he'd seen in his local paper about your doctor and breast cancer. This assumes, of course, that your search engine is aware of the Belchester Bugle website which, as we've already seen, is far from guaranteed.

Search engines do not all work the same way so a bit of trial and error is needed to work out how to get the best out of them. Some recognise certain short-cuts and not others. Search engines within a particular site – rather than a global search engine like Google – can be particularly frustrating as they have frequently not been built by search engine specialists.

How to approach the internet

The internet is a resource that can help you get the most from a consultation with a health professional. It is not a substitute for a professional consultation. These websites are listed for information only and neither the author nor the publishers can accept any responsibility for their content.

That said, don't underestimate the value of the net. In a survey in the US in 2000, 70% of patients said that information they had found on the net had influenced their health decisions. Simply remember that if you choose to do so too, it is at your own risk.

Action Cancer
Provides full-time screening clinics for women concerned about breast and cervical cancer.
Helpline. 02800 244200
Tel: 02890 803344
Fax: 02890 803356
Email: supportservices@actioncancer.org

Action On Smoking And Health (ASH)
ASH is a campaigning public health charity working for a comprehensive societal response to tobacco aimed at achieving a sharp reduction and eventual elimination of the health problems caused by tobacco.
Tel: 020 7739 5902
Fax: 020 7613 0531
Email: enquiries@ash.org.uk
Website: www.ash.org.uk

Age Concern
For up to 5 free fact sheets, or to find your local Age Concern.
Information Line: 0800 00 99 66 (7 days a week 7am–7pm)
Website: www.ageconcern.org.uk

Alcoholics Anonymous
PO Box 1
Stonebow House
Stonebow
York
YO1 7NJ
Tel: 01904 644026

American Cancer Society
The main US cancer organisation. Includes a facility for asking questions by email.
Website: www.cancer.org

Anthony Nolan Bone Marrow Trust
Searches for compatible bone marrow donors on behalf of at least 3,000 newly diagnosed patients each year. At any one time can be looking for donors for 7,000 people world-wide.
Tel: 020 7284 1234
Fax: 020 7284 8202
Email: healthgate@anthonynolan.com
Website: www.anthonynolan.org.uk

Asbestos Support Group And Mesothelioma Information Service
Helpline and other information and advice on mesothelioma (form of cancer usually caused by asbestos exposure, affecting cells lining the chest or abdominal cavities).
Tel: 0113 231 1010
Email: info@asbestos-action.org.uk
Website: www.asbestos-action.org.uk

Association for Cancer Online Resources
US-based, for people affected by cancer. Includes information and also mailing lists and discussion forums.
Website: www.acor.org

Bandolier
UK site focusing on evidence-based health care. Requires a certain amount of prior knowledge to be used effectively.
Tel: 01865 226132
Email: bandolier@pru.ox.ac.uk
Website: www.jr2.ox.ac.uk/bandolier/index.html

Beating Bowel Cancer
National bowel cancer charity.
Tel: 020 8892 5256
Fax: 020 8892 1008
Email: info@beatingbowelcancer.org
Website: www.beatingbowelcancer.org

The Bobby Moore Fund
Cancer Research UK
Raises money for research into bowel cancer and aims to raise awareness of the symptoms so that people are diagnosed earlier.
Tel: 020 7269 3412
Email: bmf@cancer.org.uk

Brain Tumour Foundation
A national organisation for patients, their families and health professionals concerned with brain tumours. Provides information, booklets and a resource library. Is developing a support network of groups and individuals.
Tel: 020 8336 2020
Email: btf.uk@virgin.net

Bristol Cancer Help Centre
Pioneer of the holistic approach to cancer care.
Helpline: 0845 123 23 10
Tel: 0117 980 9500
Fax: 0117 923 9184
Email: info@bristolcancerhelp.org
Website: www.bristolcancerhelp.org

British Acoustic Neuroma Association
Support organisation for people with acoustic neuroma run by former patients and carers.
Tel: 01623 632143
Fax: 01623 635313
Website: www.emnet.co.uk/bana/

British Association For Counselling And Psychotherapy
Provides information on training as a counsellor, as well as information on counselling services available in your locality.
Website: www.counselling.co.uk

British Colostomy Association
Support, reassurance and practical information for people with a colostomy.
Helpline: 0800 328 4257
Tel: 0118 939 1537
Fax: 0118 956 9095
Email: sue@bcass.org.uk
Website: www.bcass.org.uk

British Heart Foundation
14 Fitzhardinge Street
London
W1H 6DH
Tel: 020 7935 0185
Website: www.bhf.org.uk

Bristish Lung Foundation
The British Lung Foundation provides information on all forms of lung conditions. Runs support groups across the country.
Tel: 020 7688 5555
Fax: 020 8688 5556
Enquiries: enquiries@blf-uk.org
Website: www.britishlungfoundation.org

British Nutrition Foundation
Promotes health and well being by giving scientifically based information and advice on diet and nutrition. Cannot give individual dietary advice.
Tel: 020 7404 6504
Email: postbox@nutrition.org.uk
Website: www.nutrition.org.uk

CancerBACUP
Free cancer support service.
Freephone: 0808 800 1234
Tel: 020 7739 2280
Fax: 020 7696 9002
Website: www.cancerbacup.org.uk

Cancer Care Society

Provides free, confidential counselling, emotional support and practical help. Services include complementary therapies, befriending, an information library and a linkline for people with cancer to be put in touch with one another.
Tel: 01794 830300 (Mon-Fri 9am-5pm)

CancerHelp UK

Free service about cancer and cancer care run by Cancer Research UK. It aims to provide information on both prevention and treatment.
Email: cancer.info@cancer.org.uk
Website: www.cancerhelp.org.uk

CancerIndex

Links to cancer resources on the web by disease type and treatment. Looking up a particular type of cancer will yield a list of organisations and other resources on the web.
Website: www.cancerindex.org

Cancer Of The Eye Linkline (CELL)

24 hour helpline providing information and support for anyone who has lost an eye as a result of cancer or other trauma.
Tel: 01761 411055
Email: cell@zoom.co.uk
Website: www.cancerhelp.org.uk/ pages.zoom.co.uk/cell/index.htm

Cancer Black Care

Aims to address the cultural and emotional needs of people affected by cancer, as well as their carers, families and friends.
Tel: 020 7249 1097
Fax: 020 7249 0606
Email: cbc@cancerblackcare.org
Website: www.cancerblackcare.org/

Cancerlink

Provides emotional support and information in response to enquiries on all aspects of cancer from people with cancer, their families, friends and professionals working with them.
Helpline: 0808 808 0000

Cancer Information And Support Services

Services for cancer patients, their carers, families and friends, and for health professionals. Helpline providing information on all forms of cancer, screening, treatment and prevention.
Tel: 01792 655025
Email: cancer_info_swansea@ compuserve.com
Website: www.cancerhelp.org.uk/ www.cancerinformation.org.uk

Cancer Specialist Library (CSL)

Covers the more common cancers in details. Most useful for health professionals.
Website: www.nelc.org.uk

Cancer Support UK

This Website has been developed to provide help, support and direction for anyone living with cancer.
Website: www.cancersupportuk.nhs.uk/

Carers UK

Offer local practical and emotional support.
Tel: 0808 808 7777

Colon Cancer Concern

Dedicated to reducing deaths from bowel cancer – also known as colorectal cancer – and improving the lives of those affected by the disease.
Tel: 08708 50 60 50
Website: www.coloncancer.org.uk

Diabetes UK

10 Parkway, London, NW1 7AA
Tel: 020 7424 1030

The Digestive Disorders Foundation

Information on a wide range of digestive disorders.
Tel: 020 7486 0341
Email: ddf@digestivedisorders.org.uk
Website: www.digestivedisorders.org.uk

Drinkline

Tel: 0800 917 8282

Expert Patient Programme

Tel: 0845 606 6040
Website: www.expertpatients.nhs.uk

Family Planning Association

For advice and information on contraception, sexually transmitted infections and other sexual health issues.
2-12 Pentonville Road
London, N1 9FP
Tel: 020 7837 4044 5
Website: www.fpa.org.uk

Ileostomy and Internal Pouch Support Group

Help for people with an ileostomy or an ileo-anal pouch.
Freephone: 0800 018 4724
Email: info@the-ia.org.uk
Website: www.the-ia.org.uk

Institute For Complementary Medicine

The Institute supplies information on qualified complementary practitioners, on complementary teaching institutions and on complementary medicine generally for use by the media.
Tel: 020 7237 5165
Website: www.cmedicine.col.uk

Institute of Cancer Research

Provides links to the widely-respected Royal Marsden Hospital and its patient information section.
Website: www.icr.ac.uk/ cancerinformation.html

International Myeloma Foundation

Dedicated to improving the quality of life of Myeloma patients while working towards prevention and a cure.
Freephone: 0800 980 3332
Tel: 0131 557 3332 Fax: 0131 556 9720
Email: TheIMF@myeloma.org.uk
Website: www.myeloma.org.uk

International Stress Management Association

PO Box 348
Waltham Cross, London, EN8 8ZL
Tel: 07000 780430
Website: www.isma.org.uk

Leukaemia Care Society

Promotes the welfare of people with leukaemia and allied blood disorders; helps relieve the needs of their families.
Careline: 0800 169 6680
Tel: 01905 330003 Fax: 01905 330090
Email: admin@leukaemiacare.org
Website: www.leukaemiacare.org

Leukaemia Research Fund

Fighting leukaemia, Hodgkin's disease and other lymphomas, multiple myeloma, aplastic anaemia, myelodysplasia, the myeloproliferative disorders and related diseases.
Tel: 020 7405 0101
Email: info@lrf.org.uk
Website: www.lrf.org.uk

5

Lymphoedema Support Network

Advice and support for people suffering with lymphoedema (swelling of limbs or body due to blocked lymphatic drainage) following surgery or radiotherapy.
Tel: 020 7351 4480
Email: adminlsn@
lymphoedema.freeserve.co.uk
Website: www.lymphoedema.org

Lymphoma Association

Provides information and emotional support for lymphoma (Hodgkin's disease and non-Hodgkin's lymphoma) patients and their families.
Helpline: 0808 808 5555 (Mon-Fri, 10am-8pm)
Website: www.lymphoma.org.uk

Kidney Cancer UK

Aims to provide UK kidney cancer patients and their carers with improved access to reliable information about kidney cancer and its treatment, and to establish a network of individuals and groups capable of offering mutual support.
Helpline: 024 7647 4993 (Every day 9.30am-9.00pm)
Website: www.kcuk.org/

Macmillan

Access to publications and information about support groups, and the opportunity to read other people's stories about cancer including patients, families, friends and health professionals.
Website: www.macmillan.org.uk/
cancerinformation

MARCS Line Resource Centre

(Melanoma and Related Cancer of the Skin)
Advice line for anyone affected by melanoma or skin cancer and their families and friends. Information and advice about prevention and treatment.
Tel: 01722 415071
Website: www.wessexcancer.org
Email: marcsline@wessexcancer.org

Marie Curie Cancer Care

Marie Curie Cancer Care, the cancer care charity, provides practical hands-on nursing care at home and specialist multi-disciplinary care through its 11 Marie Curie Centres.
Tel: 020 7599 7777
Website: www.mariecurie.org.uk

The Medical Advisory Service

This organisation provides a helpline staffed by nurses. They can give you information and advice on medical problems.
Tel: 0181 994 9874 (Mon-Fri 5pm-10pm)

MedlinePLUS

General health site. The encyclopaedia section includes pictures and diagrams.
Website: medlineplus.gov

MIND (National Association for Mental Health)

Granta House
15-19 Broadway, Stratford
London, E15 4BQ
Tel: 0845 766 1063
Website: www.mind.org.uk

Move4Health

Move4Health campaigns and lobbies to make the physical, cultural, political and social environment more conducive for people being active. It also publicises how activity can promote health and wellbeing, contribute towards tackling the burden of psychological and physical disease to help reduce health inequalities in the UK.
Website: www.move4health.org.uk/

National Association for Colitis and Crohn's Disease (NACC)

For people with Crohn's disease and Colitis.
Information Line: 0845 130 2233
NACC-in-Contact Support Line: 0845 130 3344
Email: nacc@nacc.org.uk
Website: www.nacc.org.uk

National Asthma Campaign

Providence House
Providence Place
London, N1 0NT
Tel: 020 7226 2260
Fax: 020 7704 0740
Website: www.asthma.org.uk

National Cancer Alliance

National membership organisation made up of users of cancer services (patients and lay carers), health professionals and other concerned individuals or groups affected by cancer.
Tel: 01865 793566
Fax: 01865 251050
Website:
www.nationalcanceralliance.co.uk

National Obesity Forum

Established to raise awareness of the growing impact of obesity and overweight on patients and the National Health Service. Membership is open to all healthcare professionals.
Tel/Fax: 0116 8162109
Website:
www.nationalobesityforum.org.uk/
Email:
national_obesity.forum@ntlworld.com

National Osteoporosis Society

Tel: 01761 471771
Website: www.nos.org.uk

Neuroblastoma Society

Information and advice for patients and their families. Provides contact where possible with others who have experienced the illness in the family, for mutual support.
Tel: 01727 851818
Email: nsoc@ukonline.co.uk

NHS Cancer Screening Programmes

Information on bowel, breast and cervical cancer screening.
Website: www.cancerscreening.nhs.uk

NHS Direct

Website that supports the NHS Direct telephone helpline service.
Tel: 0845 46 47
Website: www.nhsdirect.nhs.uk

No Smoking Day

Whether you are a smoker who wants to give up, looking to help others to give up on No Smoking Day, or just looking for more information about the Day itself you should find everything you need here.
Tel: 0870 770 7909
Fax: 0870 770 7910
Email: enquiries@nosmokingday.org.uk

Oesophageal Patients' Association

National support organisation for oesophageal cancer patients.
Contact Mr David Kirby
Tel: 0121 704 9860

OMNI

Free access to a searchable catalogue of internet sites covering health and medicine. Possibly most useful to well-informed search engine wizards.
Website: omni.ac.uk

Oral Cancer Prevention And Detection
The Website site has detailed information about oral cancer, causes, prevention, details of examinations, presenting features, and role of the health professional.
Website:
www.gla.ac.uk/Acad/Dental/OralCancer/

OralChemo.org
An online resource for patients and their caregivers, this sites provides information on all aspects of oral chemotherapy.
Website: www.oralchemo.org

Patients' Association
Represents the views and interests of patients to government, health professionals, managers and industry and campaigns for improved health services.
Patient line: 020 8423 8999
Admin line: 020 8423 9111
Fax: 020 8423 9119

People Living with Cancer
This is the patient information site of the American Society of Clinical Oncology.
Website:
www.peoplelivingwithcancer.org

The Pituitary Foundation
Information on pituitary tumours for people diagnosed with this type of brain tumour.
Tel: 0117 927 3355

Quitline
Tel: 0800 00 22 00
Website: www.quit.org.uk

Rosemary Conley
Website:
www.rosemary-conley.co.uk

Roy Castle Lung Cancer Patient Network
A network of lung cancer information and support groups throughout the UK.
Contact Jennifer Dickson
Tel: 0800 358 7200 Fax: 01413 310590
Website: www.roycastle.org

Royal Orthopaedic Hospital Bone Tumour Service (ROHBTS for Children and Adults)
Provides support for patients with bone tumours and soft tissue tumours.
Contact Mrs Richardson
Tel: 01584 856209

The Samaritans
For emotional support for people in crisis or at risk of suicide.
Tel: 08457 90 90 90
Website: www.samaritans.org

Skinship (UK)
Helpline for people with any kind of skin problem including all types of skin cancer.
Tel: 01387 760567
Website: www.ukindex.info/skinship

Smoking helplines and websites
An advisor can put you in touch with your local NHS Stop Smoking Service.
Tel: 0800 169 0 169
Website: www.givingupsmoking.co.uk
Website: www.ash.org.uk
Website: www.sickofsmoking.com

St John Ambulance
27 St John's Lane
London, EC1M 4BU
Tel: 0870 010 4950
Website: www.sja.org.uk

TAK Tent Cancer Support
Offers support and information for cancer patients, their relatives, friends and helpers.
Helpline: 01412 110122

Tenovus Cancer Information Centre
Provides emotional support and information on all aspects of cancer for patients and their families.
Freephone Helpline: 0808 808 1010
(Mon-Fri 9am-4.30pm answerphone service)
Website: www.tenovus.org.uk

The Terrence Higgins Trust
For advice and information on HIV and AIDS.
52-54 Grays Inn Road
London
WC1 X 8JU.
Tel: 020 7242 1010
Website: www.tht.org.uk

UK Brain Tumour Society
Provides information, advice and support for anyone directly or indirectly affected by brain tumours.
Tel: 01293 781479
Fax: 01293 820720
Website: www.braintumour.org
Email: info@braintumour.org

Weight Watchers
Website: www.weightwatchers.com

WHCS Therapeutic Cancer Care
Advice, cancer care and complementary therapies for people with a diagnosis of cancer. Offer advice on cancer care, health, terminal illness, bereavement and other issues.
Tel: 0151 604 7316
Email: whcs.ttc@virgin.net
Website: www.wirralholistic.org.uk

World Cancer Research Fund
Dedicated to the prevention of cancer through healthy diets and associated lifestyles.
Website: www.wcrf-uk.org

Abdominal pain

Is the pain crushing, extending into the chest, moving to the left arm, making a sick and sweaty feeling, lasting longer than 15 minutes and not relieved by indigestion medicine (antacids)? — **YES** → **ADVICE** Call 999/112.

NO

Has a similar pain been felt more than once over the past few weeks? — **YES** → *See **Long-standing abdominal pain***

NO

Is the pain severe and is there a swollen tummy, fever or vomiting? — **YES** → **ADVICE** Call a doctor/NHS Direct.

NO

Is there a lot of blood or soil-like material in the vomit? — **YES** → **ADVICE** Call 999/112.

NO

Is there tar-like material or blood in the bowel motions? — **YES** → **ADVICE** Call a doctor/NHS Direct.

NO

Is there diarrhoea? — **YES** → *See **Diarrhoea*** **ADVICE** Diarrhoea can be caused by some medicines such as antibiotics. Ask a pharmacist about any medicines being taken. If there is also severe pain or vomiting it may mean food poisoning. Call a doctor/NHS Direct.

NO

Is the pain also moving to the groin? — **YES** → *See **Urinary problems*** **ADVICE** May be an infection of the kidney or a kidney stone. If there is no relief with paracetamol or the pain is very severe, call a doctor/NHS Direct.

NO

Could the sufferer be pregnant? — **YES** → **ADVICE** Call a doctor/NHS Direct.

NO

H45179

Abdominal pain

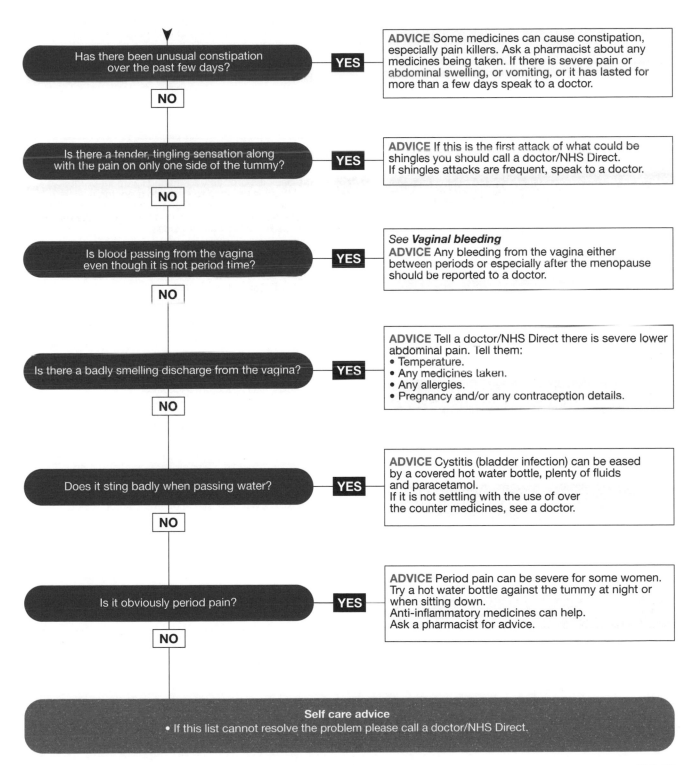

Has there been unusual constipation over the past few days? **YES** → **ADVICE** Some medicines can cause constipation, especially pain killers. Ask a pharmacist about any medicines being taken. If there is severe pain or abdominal swelling, or vomiting, or it has lasted for more than a few days speak to a doctor.

NO

Is there a tender, tingling sensation along with the pain on only one side of the tummy? **YES** → **ADVICE** If this is the first attack of what could be shingles you should call a doctor/NHS Direct. If shingles attacks are frequent, speak to a doctor.

NO

Is blood passing from the vagina even though it is not period time? **YES** → See *Vaginal bleeding* **ADVICE** Any bleeding from the vagina either between periods or especially after the menopause should be reported to a doctor.

NO

Is there a badly smelling discharge from the vagina? **YES** → **ADVICE** Tell a doctor/NHS Direct there is severe lower abdominal pain. Tell them:
• Temperature.
• Any medicines taken.
• Any allergies.
• Pregnancy and/or any contraception details.

NO

Does it sting badly when passing water? **YES** → **ADVICE** Cystitis (bladder infection) can be eased by a covered hot water bottle, plenty of fluids and paracetamol. If it is not settling with the use of over the counter medicines, see a doctor.

NO

Is it obviously period pain? **YES** → **ADVICE** Period pain can be severe for some women. Try a hot water bottle against the tummy at night or when sitting down. Anti-inflammatory medicines can help. Ask a pharmacist for advice.

NO

Self care advice
• If this list cannot resolve the problem please call a doctor/NHS Direct.

H45180

Backache

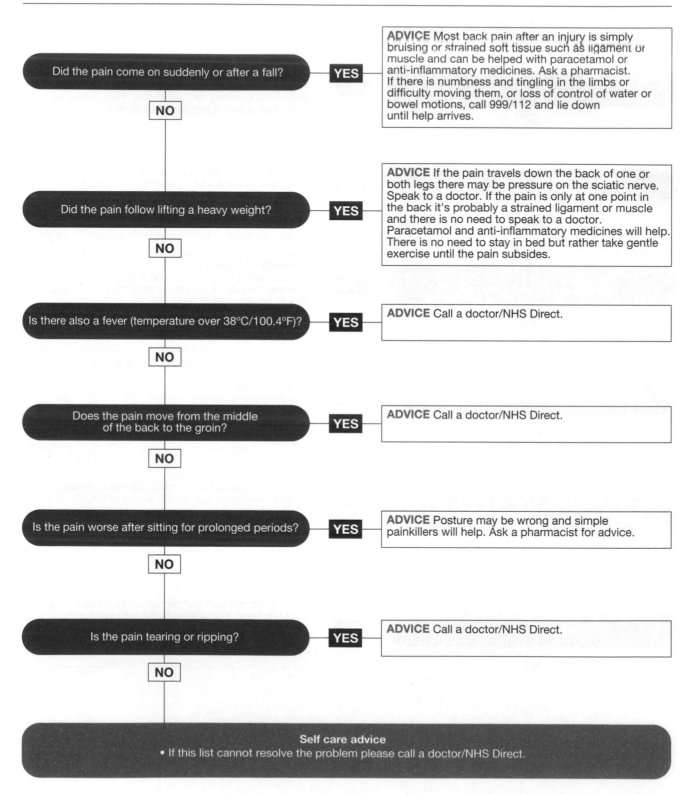

Did the pain come on suddenly or after a fall? — **YES**

ADVICE Most back pain after an injury is simply bruising or strained soft tissue such as ligament or muscle and can be helped with paracetamol or anti-inflammatory medicines. Ask a pharmacist. If there is numbness and tingling in the limbs or difficulty moving them, or loss of control of water or bowel motions, call 999/112 and lie down until help arrives.

NO

Did the pain follow lifting a heavy weight? — **YES**

ADVICE If the pain travels down the back of one or both legs there may be pressure on the sciatic nerve. Speak to a doctor. If the pain is only at one point in the back it's probably a strained ligament or muscle and there is no need to speak to a doctor. Paracetamol and anti-inflammatory medicines will help. There is no need to stay in bed but rather take gentle exercise until the pain subsides.

NO

Is there also a fever (temperature over 38°C/100.4°F)? — **YES**

ADVICE Call a doctor/NHS Direct.

NO

Does the pain move from the middle of the back to the groin? — **YES**

ADVICE Call a doctor/NHS Direct.

NO

Is the pain worse after sitting for prolonged periods? — **YES**

ADVICE Posture may be wrong and simple painkillers will help. Ask a pharmacist for advice.

NO

Is the pain tearing or ripping? — **YES**

ADVICE Call a doctor/NHS Direct.

NO

Self care advice
• If this list cannot resolve the problem please call a doctor/NHS Direct.

H45181

Breast changes

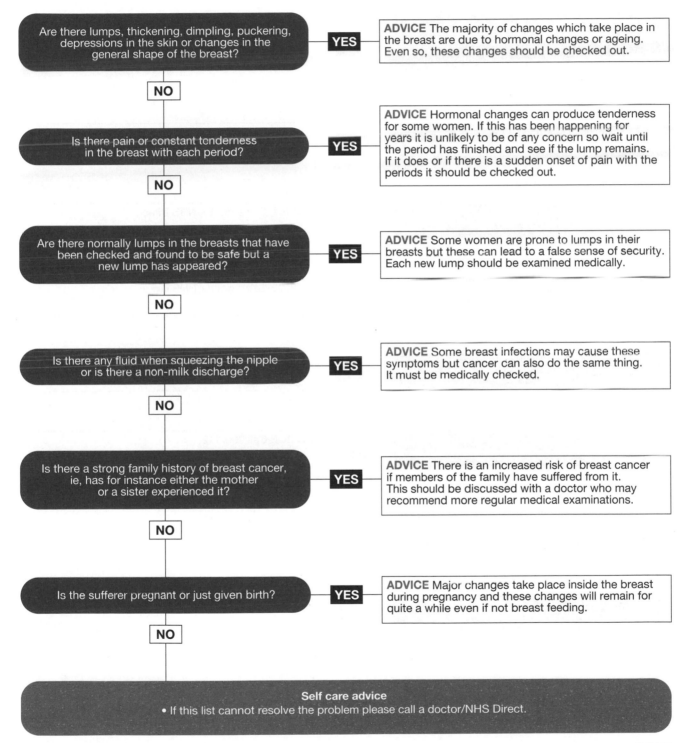

Are there lumps, thickening, dimpling, puckering, depressions in the skin or changes in the general shape of the breast?

YES — ADVICE The majority of changes which take place in the breast are due to hormonal changes or ageing. Even so, these changes should be checked out.

NO

Is there pain or constant tenderness in the breast with each period?

YES — ADVICE Hormonal changes can produce tenderness for some women. If this has been happening for years it is unlikely to be of any concern so wait until the period has finished and see if the lump remains. If it does or if there is a sudden onset of pain with the periods it should be checked out.

NO

Are there normally lumps in the breasts that have been checked and found to be safe but a new lump has appeared?

YES — ADVICE Some women are prone to lumps in their breasts but these can lead to a false sense of security. Each new lump should be examined medically.

NO

Is there any fluid when squeezing the nipple or is there a non-milk discharge?

YES — ADVICE Some breast infections may cause these symptoms but cancer can also do the same thing. It must be medically checked.

NO

Is there a strong family history of breast cancer, ie, has for instance either the mother or a sister experienced it?

YES — ADVICE There is an increased risk of breast cancer if members of the family have suffered from it. This should be discussed with a doctor who may recommend more regular medical examinations.

NO

Is the sufferer pregnant or just given birth?

YES — ADVICE Major changes take place inside the breast during pregnancy and these changes will remain for quite a while even if not breast feeding.

NO

Self care advice
• If this list cannot resolve the problem please call a doctor/NHS Direct.

H45182

Breathing difficulty

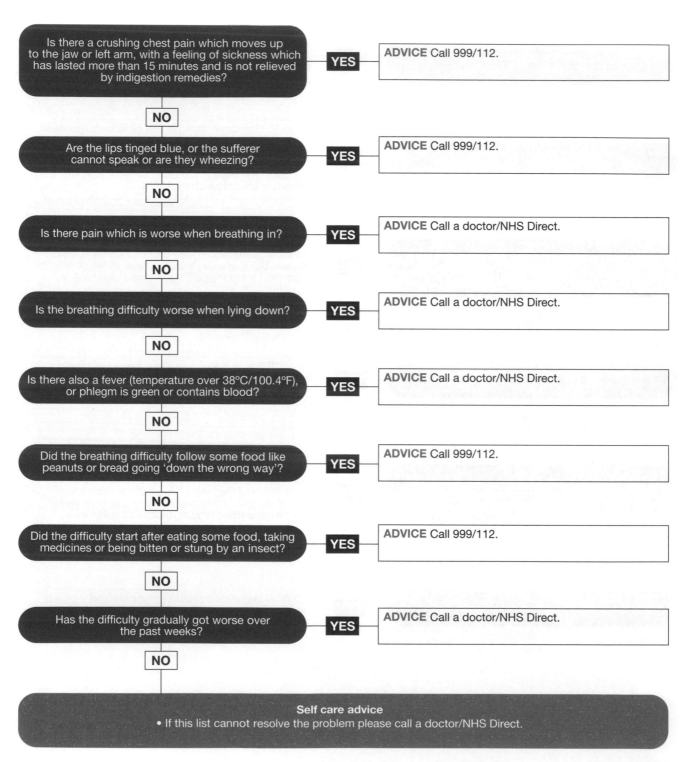

Is there a crushing chest pain which moves up to the jaw or left arm, with a feeling of sickness which has lasted more than 15 minutes and is not relieved by indigestion remedies?

YES → **ADVICE** Call 999/112.

NO

Are the lips tinged blue, or the sufferer cannot speak or are they wheezing?

YES → **ADVICE** Call 999/112.

NO

Is there pain which is worse when breathing in?

YES → **ADVICE** Call a doctor/NHS Direct.

NO

Is the breathing difficulty worse when lying down?

YES → **ADVICE** Call a doctor/NHS Direct.

NO

Is there also a fever (temperature over 38°C/100.4°F), or phlegm is green or contains blood?

YES → **ADVICE** Call a doctor/NHS Direct.

NO

Did the breathing difficulty follow some food like peanuts or bread going 'down the wrong way'?

YES → **ADVICE** Call 999/112.

NO

Did the difficulty start after eating some food, taking medicines or being bitten or stung by an insect?

YES → **ADVICE** Call 999/112.

NO

Has the difficulty gradually got worse over the past weeks?

YES → **ADVICE** Call a doctor/NHS Direct.

NO

Self care advice
• If this list cannot resolve the problem please call a doctor/NHS Direct.

H45183

Chest pain

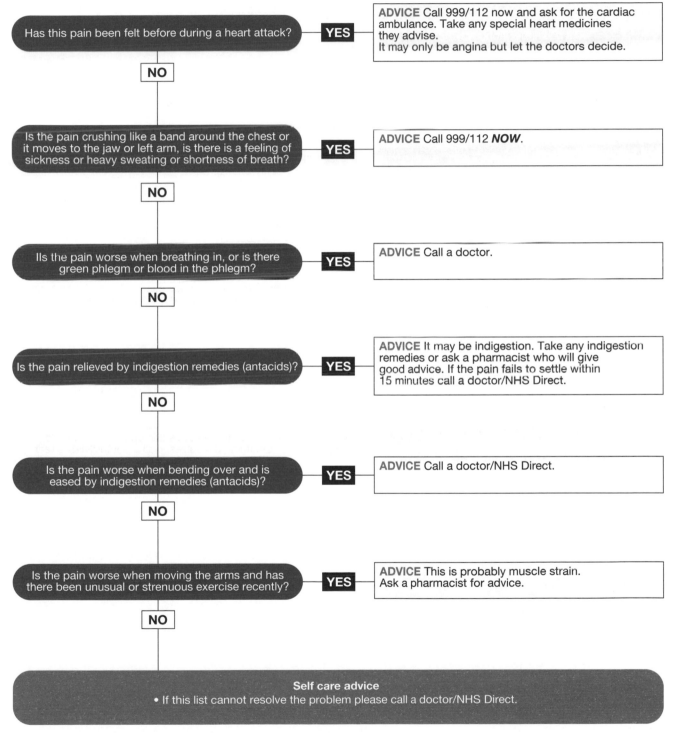

Has this pain been felt before during a heart attack?

YES → **ADVICE** Call 999/112 now and ask for the cardiac ambulance. Take any special heart medicines they advise.
It may only be angina but let the doctors decide.

NO

Is the pain crushing like a band around the chest or it moves to the jaw or left arm, is there is a feeling of sickness or heavy sweating or shortness of breath?

YES → **ADVICE** Call 999/112 *NOW*.

NO

Ils the pain worse when breathing in, or is there green phlegm or blood in the phlegm?

YES → **ADVICE** Call a doctor.

NO

Is the pain relieved by indigestion remedies (antacids)?

YES → **ADVICE** It may be indigestion. Take any indigestion remedies or ask a pharmacist who will give good advice. If the pain fails to settle within 15 minutes call a doctor/NHS Direct.

NO

Is the pain worse when bending over and is eased by indigestion remedies (antacids)?

YES → **ADVICE** Call a doctor/NHS Direct.

NO

Is the pain worse when moving the arms and has there been unusual or strenuous exercise recently?

YES → **ADVICE** This is probably muscle strain.
Ask a pharmacist for advice.

NO

Self care advice
• If this list cannot resolve the problem please call a doctor/NHS Direct.

H45184

Coughing

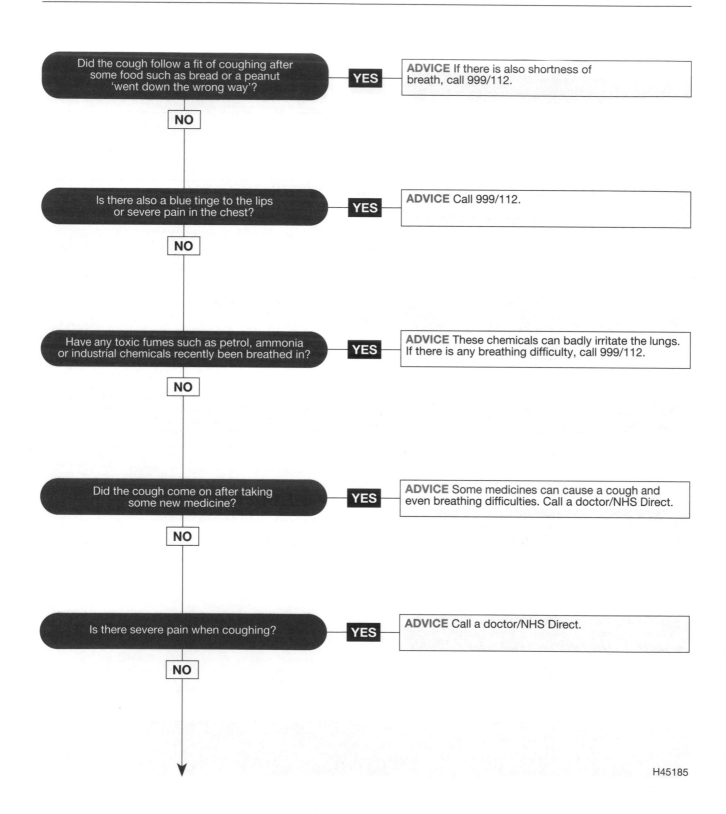

Did the cough follow a fit of coughing after some food such as bread or a peanut 'went down the wrong way'?

YES → ADVICE If there is also shortness of breath, call 999/112.

NO

Is there also a blue tinge to the lips or severe pain in the chest?

YES → ADVICE Call 999/112.

NO

Have any toxic fumes such as petrol, ammonia or industrial chemicals recently been breathed in?

YES → ADVICE These chemicals can badly irritate the lungs. If there is any breathing difficulty, call 999/112.

NO

Did the cough come on after taking some new medicine?

YES → ADVICE Some medicines can cause a cough and even breathing difficulties. Call a doctor/NHS Direct.

NO

Is there severe pain when coughing?

YES → ADVICE Call a doctor/NHS Direct.

NO

H45185

Coughing

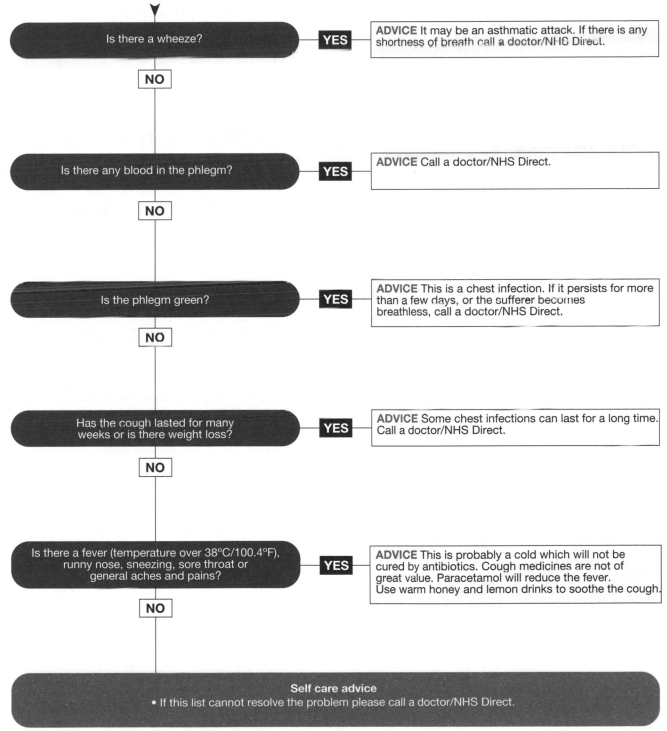

Is there a wheeze? **YES** **ADVICE** It may be an asthmatic attack. If there is any shortness of breath call a doctor/NHS Direct.

NO

Is there any blood in the phlegm? **YES** **ADVICE** Call a doctor/NHS Direct.

NO

Is the phlegm green? **YES** **ADVICE** This is a chest infection. If it persists for more than a few days, or the sufferer becomes breathless, call a doctor/NHS Direct.

NO

Has the cough lasted for many weeks or is there weight loss? **YES** **ADVICE** Some chest infections can last for a long time. Call a doctor/NHS Direct.

NO

Is there a fever (temperature over 38°C/100.4°F), runny nose, sneezing, sore throat or general aches and pains? **YES** **ADVICE** This is probably a cold which will not be cured by antibiotics. Cough medicines are not of great value. Paracetamol will reduce the fever. Use warm honey and lemon drinks to soothe the cough.

NO

Self care advice
• If this list cannot resolve the problem please call a doctor/NHS Direct.

H45186

Depression

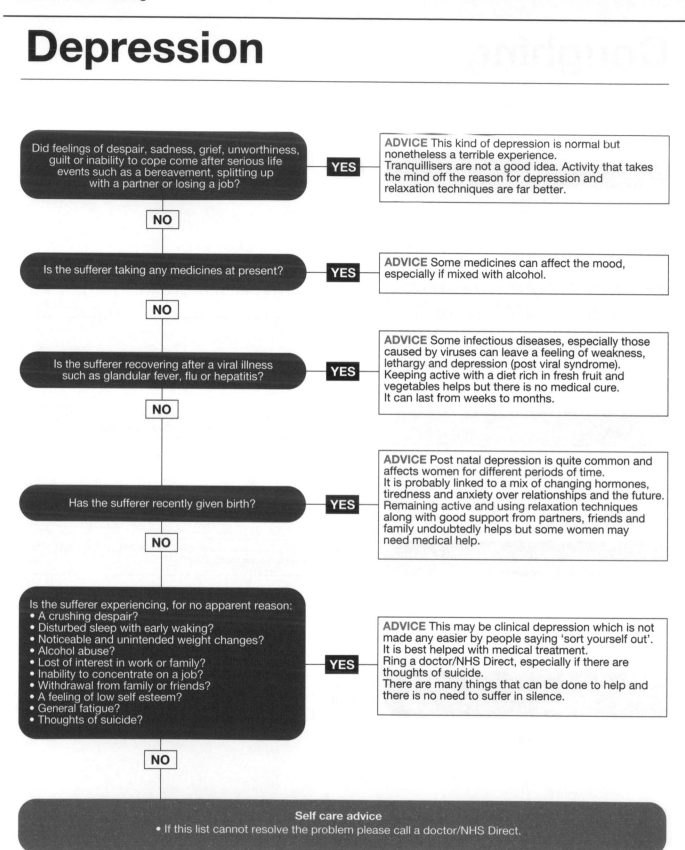

Did feelings of despair, sadness, grief, unworthiness, guilt or inability to cope come after serious life events such as a bereavement, splitting up with a partner or losing a job?

YES — **ADVICE** This kind of depression is normal but nonetheless a terrible experience. Tranquillisers are not a good idea. Activity that takes the mind off the reason for depression and relaxation techniques are far better.

NO

Is the sufferer taking any medicines at present?

YES — **ADVICE** Some medicines can affect the mood, especially if mixed with alcohol.

NO

Is the sufferer recovering after a viral illness such as glandular fever, flu or hepatitis?

YES — **ADVICE** Some infectious diseases, especially those caused by viruses can leave a feeling of weakness, lethargy and depression (post viral syndrome). Keeping active with a diet rich in fresh fruit and vegetables helps but there is no medical cure. It can last from weeks to months.

NO

Has the sufferer recently given birth?

YES — **ADVICE** Post natal depression is quite common and affects women for different periods of time. It is probably linked to a mix of changing hormones, tiredness and anxiety over relationships and the future. Remaining active and using relaxation techniques along with good support from partners, friends and family undoubtedly helps but some women may need medical help.

NO

Is the sufferer experiencing, for no apparent reason:
• A crushing despair?
• Disturbed sleep with early waking?
• Noticeable and unintended weight changes?
• Alcohol abuse?
• Lost of interest in work or family?
• Inability to concentrate on a job?
• Withdrawal from family or friends?
• A feeling of low self esteem?
• General fatigue?
• Thoughts of suicide?

YES — **ADVICE** This may be clinical depression which is not made any easier by people saying 'sort yourself out'. It is best helped with medical treatment. Ring a doctor/NHS Direct, especially if there are thoughts of suicide. There are many things that can be done to help and there is no need to suffer in silence.

NO

Self care advice
• If this list cannot resolve the problem please call a doctor/NHS Direct.

H45187

Diarrhoea

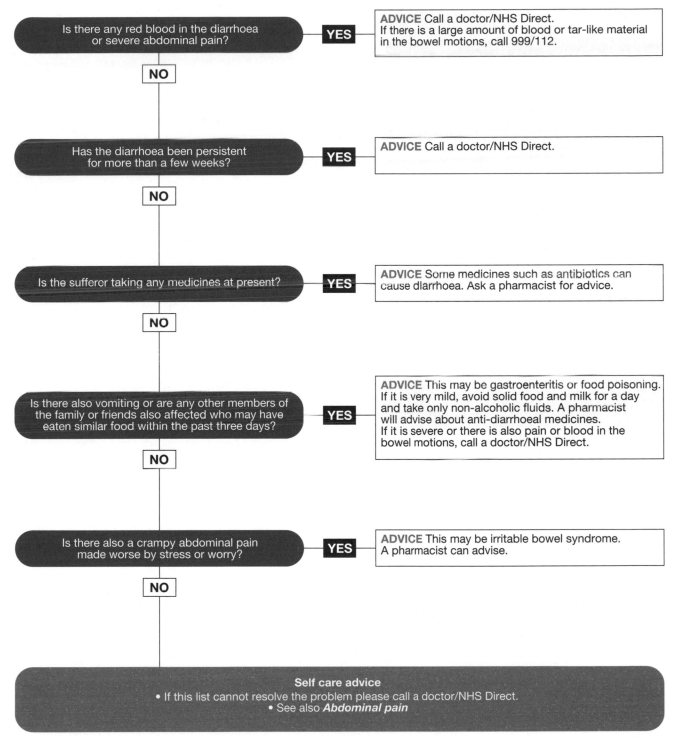

Is there any red blood in the diarrhoea or severe abdominal pain?

YES → **ADVICE** Call a doctor/NHS Direct.
If there is a large amount of blood or tar-like material in the bowel motions, call 999/112.

NO ↓

Has the diarrhoea been persistent for more than a few weeks?

YES → **ADVICE** Call a doctor/NHS Direct.

NO ↓

Is the sufferer taking any medicines at present?

YES → **ADVICE** Some medicines such as antibiotics can cause diarrhoea. Ask a pharmacist for advice.

NO ↓

Is there also vomiting or are any other members of the family or friends also affected who may have eaten similar food within the past three days?

YES → **ADVICE** This may be gastroenteritis or food poisoning. If it is very mild, avoid solid food and milk for a day and take only non-alcoholic fluids. A pharmacist will advise about anti-diarrhoeal medicines.
If it is severe or there is also pain or blood in the bowel motions, call a doctor/NHS Direct.

NO ↓

Is there also a crampy abdominal pain made worse by stress or worry?

YES → **ADVICE** This may be irritable bowel syndrome. A pharmacist can advise.

NO ↓

Self care advice
• If this list cannot resolve the problem please call a doctor/NHS Direct.
• See also *Abdominal pain*

H45188

Fever

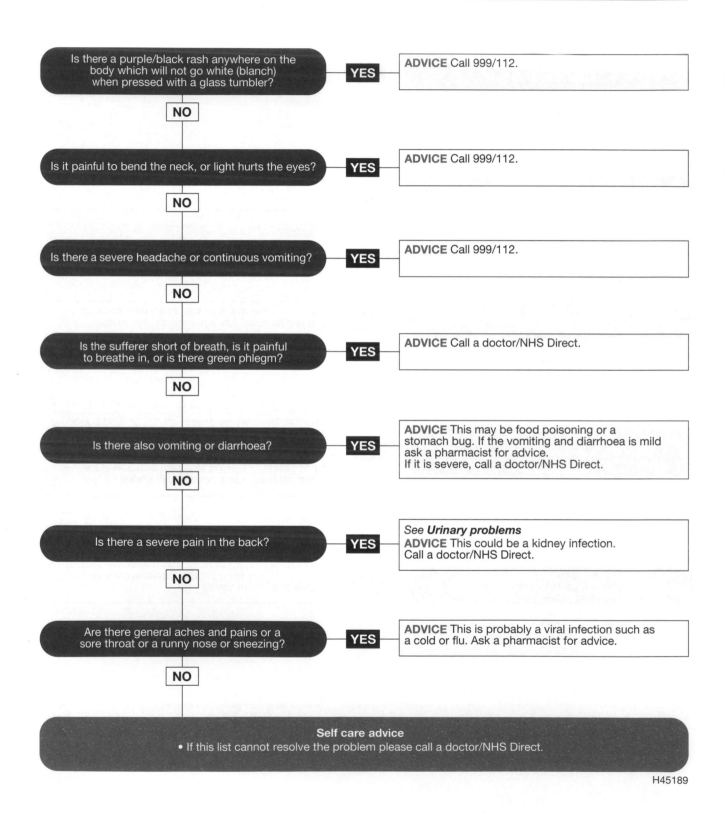

Is there a purple/black rash anywhere on the body which will not go white (blanch) when pressed with a glass tumbler?

YES → **ADVICE** Call 999/112.

NO

Is it painful to bend the neck, or light hurts the eyes?

YES → **ADVICE** Call 999/112.

NO

Is there a severe headache or continuous vomiting?

YES → **ADVICE** Call 999/112.

NO

Is the sufferer short of breath, is it painful to breathe in, or is there green phlegm?

YES → **ADVICE** Call a doctor/NHS Direct.

NO

Is there also vomiting or diarrhoea?

YES → **ADVICE** This may be food poisoning or a stomach bug. If the vomiting and diarrhoea is mild ask a pharmacist for advice.
If it is severe, call a doctor/NHS Direct.

NO

Is there a severe pain in the back?

YES → See ***Urinary problems***
ADVICE This could be a kidney infection. Call a doctor/NHS Direct.

NO

Are there general aches and pains or a sore throat or a runny nose or sneezing?

YES → **ADVICE** This is probably a viral infection such as a cold or flu. Ask a pharmacist for advice.

NO

Self care advice
• If this list cannot resolve the problem please call a doctor/NHS Direct.

H45189

Headaches

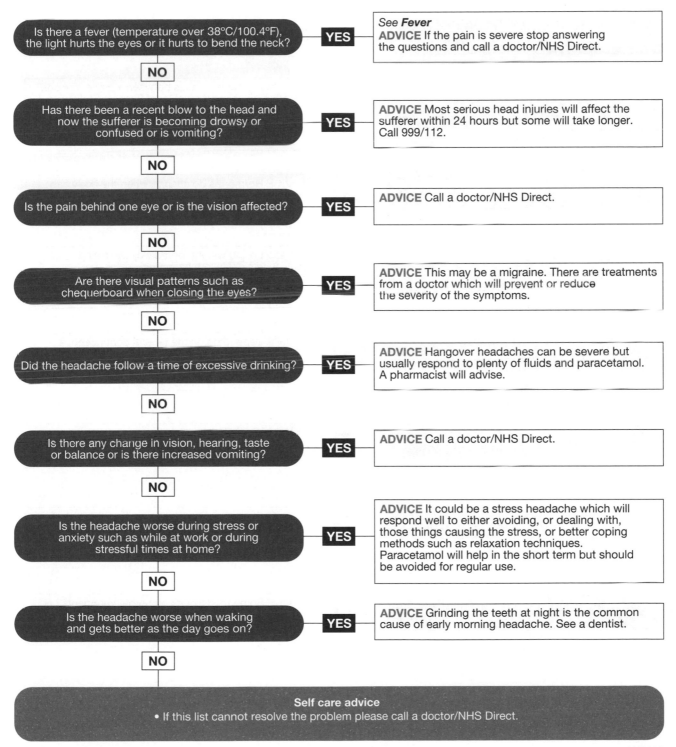

Is there a fever (temperature over 38°C/100.4°F), the light hurts the eyes or it hurts to bend the neck?

YES

*See **Fever***
ADVICE If the pain is severe stop answering the questions and call a doctor/NHS Direct.

NO

Has there been a recent blow to the head and now the sufferer is becoming drowsy or confused or is vomiting?

YES

ADVICE Most serious head injuries will affect the sufferer within 24 hours but some will take longer. Call 999/112.

NO

Is the pain behind one eye or is the vision affected?

YES

ADVICE Call a doctor/NHS Direct.

NO

Are there visual patterns such as chequerboard when closing the eyes?

YES

ADVICE This may be a migraine. There are treatments from a doctor which will prevent or reduce the severity of the symptoms.

NO

Did the headache follow a time of excessive drinking?

YES

ADVICE Hangover headaches can be severe but usually respond to plenty of fluids and paracetamol. A pharmacist will advise.

NO

Is there any change in vision, hearing, taste or balance or is there increased vomiting?

YES

ADVICE Call a doctor/NHS Direct.

NO

Is the headache worse during stress or anxiety such as while at work or during stressful times at home?

YES

ADVICE It could be a stress headache which will respond well to either avoiding, or dealing with, those things causing the stress, or better coping methods such as relaxation techniques. Paracetamol will help in the short term but should be avoided for regular use.

NO

Is the headache worse when waking and gets better as the day goes on?

YES

ADVICE Grinding the teeth at night is the common cause of early morning headache. See a dentist.

NO

Self care advice
• If this list cannot resolve the problem please call a doctor/NHS Direct.

H45190

Irregular periods

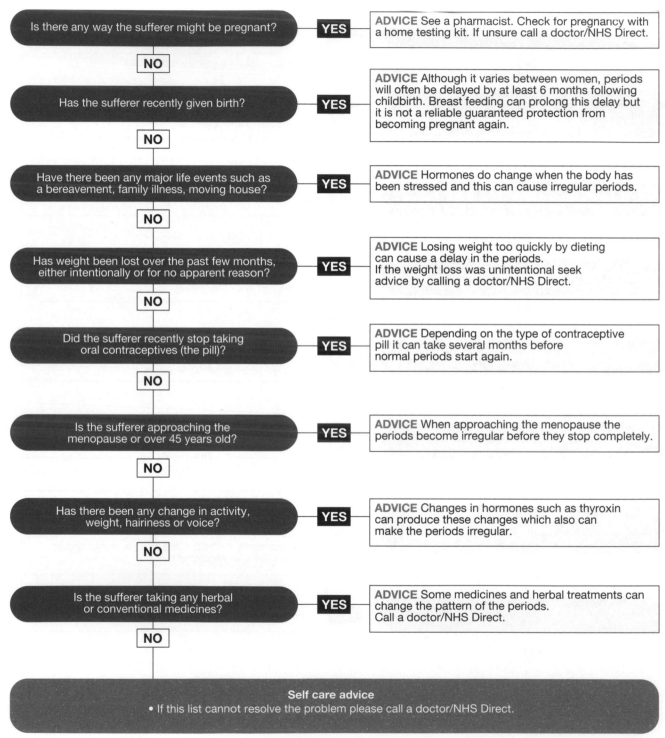

Is there any way the sufferer might be pregnant? **YES** ADVICE See a pharmacist. Check for pregnancy with a home testing kit. If unsure call a doctor/NHS Direct.

NO

Has the sufferer recently given birth? **YES** ADVICE Although it varies between women, periods will often be delayed by at least 6 months following childbirth. Breast feeding can prolong this delay but it is not a reliable guaranteed protection from becoming pregnant again.

NO

Have there been any major life events such as a bereavement, family illness, moving house? **YES** ADVICE Hormones do change when the body has been stressed and this can cause irregular periods.

NO

Has weight been lost over the past few months, either intentionally or for no apparent reason? **YES** ADVICE Losing weight too quickly by dieting can cause a delay in the periods. If the weight loss was unintentional seek advice by calling a doctor/NHS Direct.

NO

Did the sufferer recently stop taking oral contraceptives (the pill)? **YES** ADVICE Depending on the type of contraceptive pill it can take several months before normal periods start again.

NO

Is the sufferer approaching the menopause or over 45 years old? **YES** ADVICE When approaching the menopause the periods become irregular before they stop completely.

NO

Has there been any change in activity, weight, hairiness or voice? **YES** ADVICE Changes in hormones such as thyroxin can produce these changes which also can make the periods irregular.

NO

Is the sufferer taking any herbal or conventional medicines? **YES** ADVICE Some medicines and herbal treatments can change the pattern of the periods. Call a doctor/NHS Direct.

NO

Self care advice
• If this list cannot resolve the problem please call a doctor/NHS Direct.

H45191

Joint pain

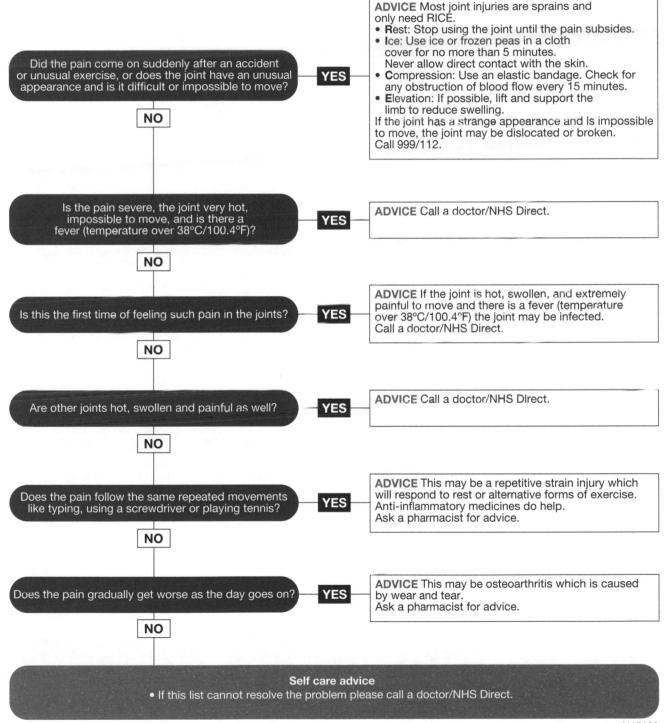

Did the pain come on suddenly after an accident or unusual exercise, or does the joint have an unusual appearance and is it difficult or impossible to move?

YES

ADVICE Most joint injuries are sprains and only need RICE.
- **R**est: Stop using the joint until the pain subsides.
- **I**ce: Use ice or frozen peas in a cloth cover for no more than 5 minutes. Never allow direct contact with the skin.
- **C**ompression: Use an elastic bandage. Check for any obstruction of blood flow every 15 minutes.
- **E**levation: If possible, lift and support the limb to reduce swelling.

If the joint has a strange appearance and is impossible to move, the joint may be dislocated or broken. Call 999/112.

NO

Is the pain severe, the joint very hot, impossible to move, and is there a fever (temperature over 38°C/100.4°F)?

YES

ADVICE Call a doctor/NHS Direct.

NO

Is this the first time of feeling such pain in the joints?

YES

ADVICE If the joint is hot, swollen, and extremely painful to move and there is a fever (temperature over 38°C/100.4°F) the joint may be infected. Call a doctor/NHS Direct.

NO

Are other joints hot, swollen and painful as well?

YES

ADVICE Call a doctor/NHS Direct.

NO

Does the pain follow the same repeated movements like typing, using a screwdriver or playing tennis?

YES

ADVICE This may be a repetitive strain injury which will respond to rest or alternative forms of exercise. Anti-inflammatory medicines do help. Ask a pharmacist for advice.

NO

Does the pain gradually get worse as the day goes on?

YES

ADVICE This may be osteoarthritis which is caused by wear and tear. Ask a pharmacist for advice.

NO

Self care advice
- If this list cannot resolve the problem please call a doctor/NHS Direct.

H45192

Long-standing abdominal pain

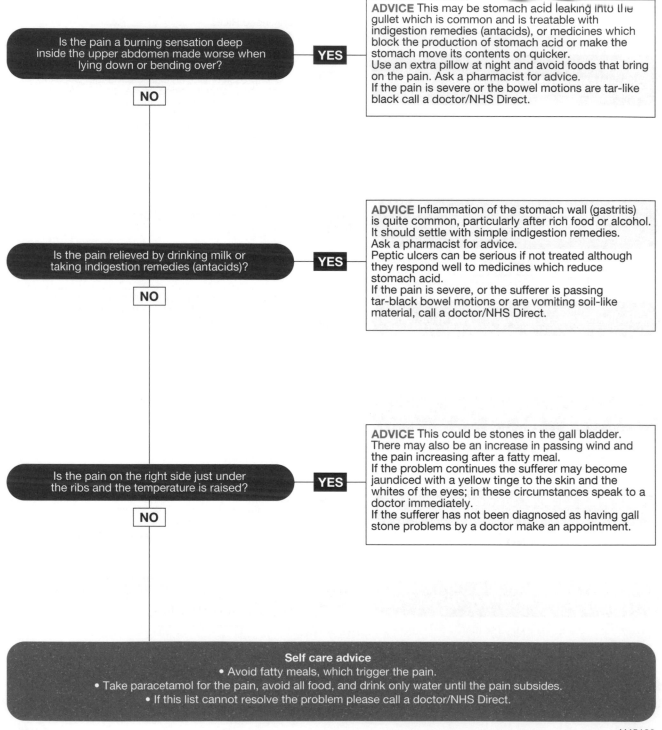

Is the pain a burning sensation deep inside the upper abdomen made worse when lying down or bending over?

YES

ADVICE This may be stomach acid leaking into the gullet which is common and is treatable with indigestion remedies (antacids), or medicines which block the production of stomach acid or make the stomach move its contents on quicker.
Use an extra pillow at night and avoid foods that bring on the pain. Ask a pharmacist for advice.
If the pain is severe or the bowel motions are tar-like black call a doctor/NHS Direct.

NO

Is the pain relieved by drinking milk or taking indigestion remedies (antacids)?

YES

ADVICE Inflammation of the stomach wall (gastritis) is quite common, particularly after rich food or alcohol. It should settle with simple indigestion remedies. Ask a pharmacist for advice.
Peptic ulcers can be serious if not treated although they respond well to medicines which reduce stomach acid.
If the pain is severe, or the sufferer is passing tar-black bowel motions or are vomiting soil-like material, call a doctor/NHS Direct.

NO

Is the pain on the right side just under the ribs and the temperature is raised?

YES

ADVICE This could be stones in the gall bladder. There may also be an increase in passing wind and the pain increasing after a fatty meal.
If the problem continues the sufferer may become jaundiced with a yellow tinge to the skin and the whites of the eyes; in these circumstances speak to a doctor immediately.
If the sufferer has not been diagnosed as having gall stone problems by a doctor make an appointment.

NO

Self care advice
• Avoid fatty meals, which trigger the pain.
• Take paracetamol for the pain, avoid all food, and drink only water until the pain subsides.
• If this list cannot resolve the problem please call a doctor/NHS Direct.

H45193

Stress

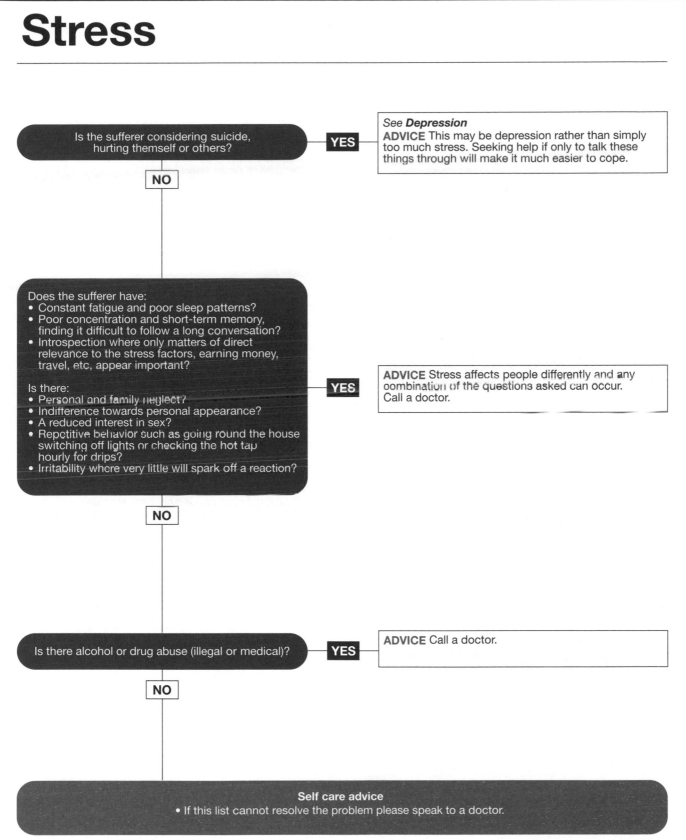

Is the sufferer considering suicide, hurting themself or others?

YES

*See **Depression***
ADVICE This may be depression rather than simply too much stress. Seeking help if only to talk these things through will make it much easier to cope.

NO

Does the sufferer have:
• Constant fatigue and poor sleep patterns?
• Poor concentration and short-term memory, finding it difficult to follow a long conversation?
• Introspection where only matters of direct relevance to the stress factors, earning money, travel, etc, appear important?

Is there:
• Personal and family neglect?
• Indifference towards personal appearance?
• A reduced interest in sex?
• Repetitive behavior such as going round the house switching off lights or checking the hot tap hourly for drips?
• Irritability where very little will spark off a reaction?

YES

ADVICE Stress affects people differently and any combination of the questions asked can occur. Call a doctor.

NO

Is there alcohol or drug abuse (illegal or medical)?

YES

ADVICE Call a doctor.

NO

Self care advice
• If this list cannot resolve the problem please speak to a doctor.

H45194

Vaginal bleeding

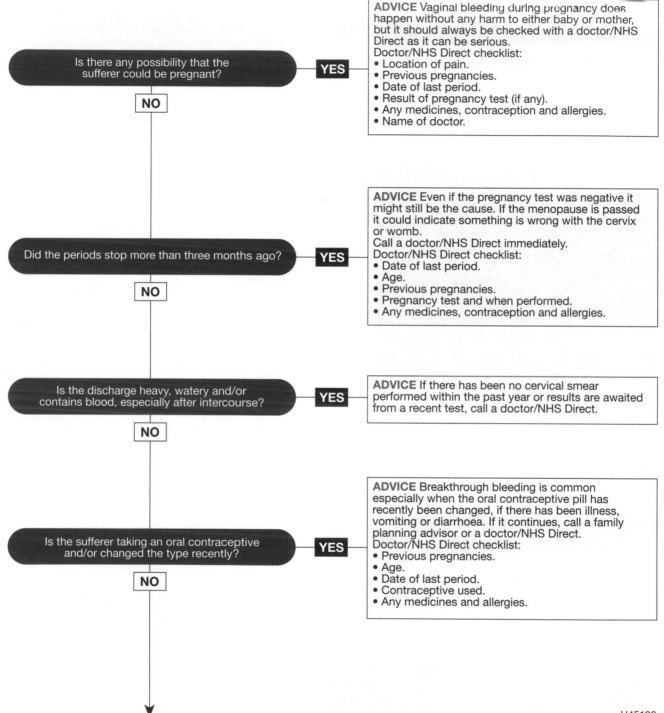

Is there any possibility that the sufferer could be pregnant?

YES — **ADVICE** Vaginal bleeding during pregnancy does happen without any harm to either baby or mother, but it should always be checked with a doctor/NHS Direct as it can be serious.
Doctor/NHS Direct checklist:
• Location of pain.
• Previous pregnancies.
• Date of last period.
• Result of pregnancy test (if any).
• Any medicines, contraception and allergies.
• Name of doctor.

NO

Did the periods stop more than three months ago?

YES — **ADVICE** Even if the pregnancy test was negative it might still be the cause. If the menopause is passed it could indicate something is wrong with the cervix or womb.
Call a doctor/NHS Direct immediately.
Doctor/NHS Direct checklist:
• Date of last period.
• Age.
• Previous pregnancies.
• Pregnancy test and when performed.
• Any medicines, contraception and allergies.

NO

Is the discharge heavy, watery and/or contains blood, especially after intercourse?

YES — **ADVICE** If there has been no cervical smear performed within the past year or results are awaited from a recent test, call a doctor/NHS Direct.

NO

Is the sufferer taking an oral contraceptive and/or changed the type recently?

YES — **ADVICE** Breakthrough bleeding is common especially when the oral contraceptive pill has recently been changed, if there has been illness, vomiting or diarrhoea. If it continues, call a family planning advisor or a doctor/NHS Direct.
Doctor/NHS Direct checklist:
• Previous pregnancies.
• Age.
• Date of last period.
• Contraceptive used.
• Any medicines and allergies.

NO

H45196

Vaginal bleeding

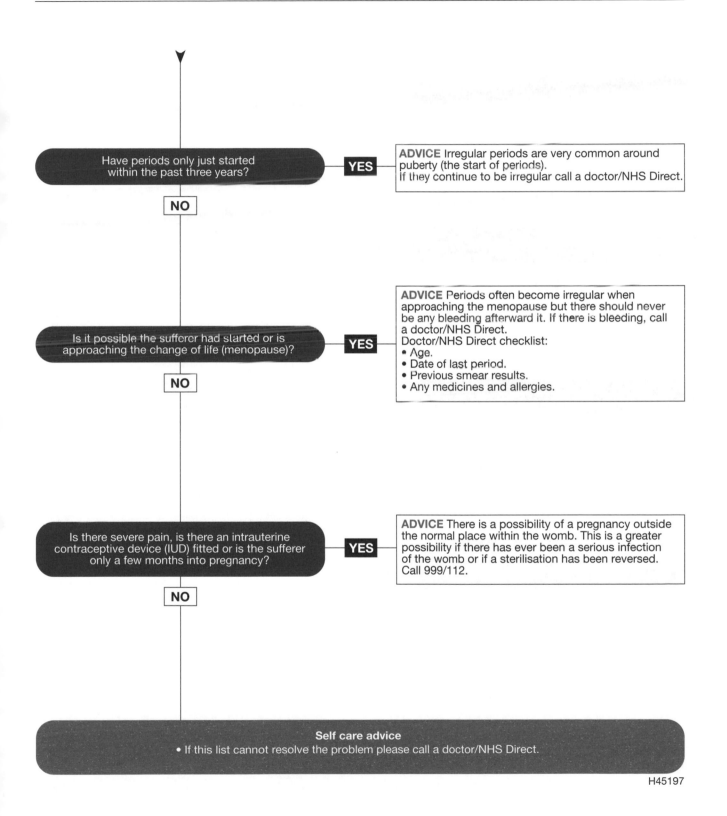

Have periods only just started within the past three years?

YES

ADVICE Irregular periods are very common around puberty (the start of periods).
If they continue to be irregular call a doctor/NHS Direct.

NO

Is it possible the sufferer had started or is approaching the change of life (menopause)?

YES

ADVICE Periods often become irregular when approaching the menopause but there should never be any bleeding afterward it. If there is bleeding, call a doctor/NHS Direct.
Doctor/NHS Direct checklist:
• Age.
• Date of last period.
• Previous smear results.
• Any medicines and allergies.

NO

Is there severe pain, is there an intrauterine contraceptive device (IUD) fitted or is the sufferer only a few months into pregnancy?

YES

ADVICE There is a possibility of a pregnancy outside the normal place within the womb. This is a greater possibility if there has ever been a serious infection of the womb or if a sterilisation has been reversed. Call 999/112.

NO

Self care advice
• If this list cannot resolve the problem please call a doctor/NHS Direct.

H45197

Urinary problems

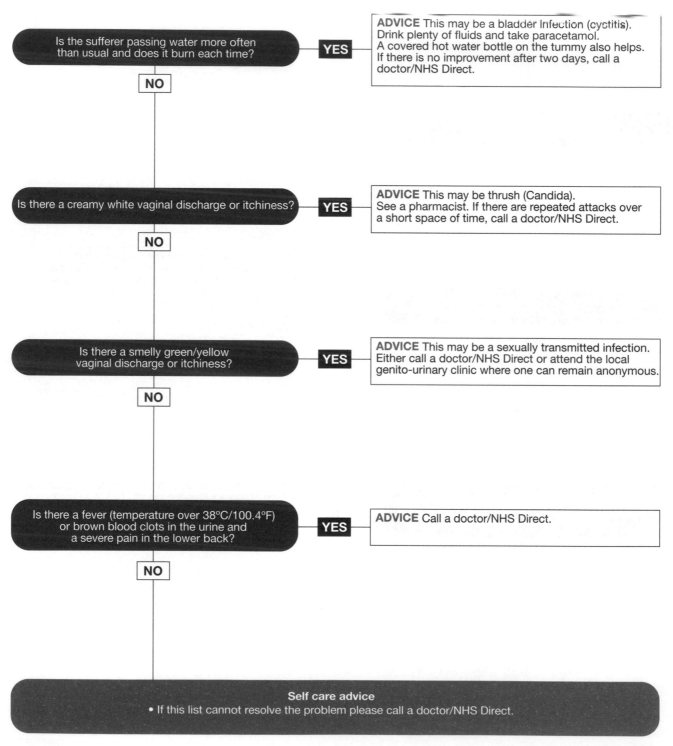

Is the sufferer passing water more often than usual and does it burn each time?

YES — **ADVICE** This may be a bladder infection (cystitis). Drink plenty of fluids and take paracetamol. A covered hot water bottle on the tummy also helps. If there is no improvement after two days, call a doctor/NHS Direct.

NO

Is there a creamy white vaginal discharge or itchiness?

YES — **ADVICE** This may be thrush (Candida). See a pharmacist. If there are repeated attacks over a short space of time, call a doctor/NHS Direct.

NO

Is there a smelly green/yellow vaginal discharge or itchiness?

YES — **ADVICE** This may be a sexually transmitted infection. Either call a doctor/NHS Direct or attend the local genito-urinary clinic where one can remain anonymous.

NO

Is there a fever (temperature over 38°C/100.4°F) or brown blood clots in the urine and a severe pain in the lower back?

YES — **ADVICE** Call a doctor/NHS Direct.

NO

Self care advice
• If this list cannot resolve the problem please call a doctor/NHS Direct.

H45195

Weight loss (without dieting or trying to lose weight)

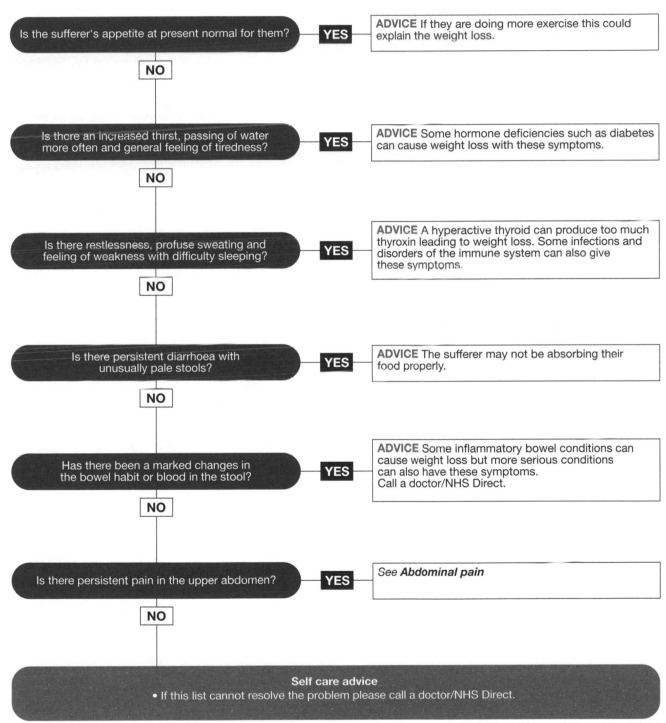

Is the sufferer's appetite at present normal for them?
YES ADVICE If they are doing more exercise this could explain the weight loss.

NO

Is there an increased thirst, passing of water more often and general feeling of tiredness?
YES ADVICE Some hormone deficiencies such as diabetes can cause weight loss with these symptoms.

NO

Is there restlessness, profuse sweating and feeling of weakness with difficulty sleeping?
YES ADVICE A hyperactive thyroid can produce too much thyroxin leading to weight loss. Some infections and disorders of the immune system can also give these symptoms.

NO

Is there persistent diarrhoea with unusually pale stools?
YES ADVICE The sufferer may not be absorbing their food properly.

NO

Has there been a marked changes in the bowel habit or blood in the stool?
YES ADVICE Some inflammatory bowel conditions can cause weight loss but more serious conditions can also have these symptoms. Call a doctor/NHS Direct.

NO

Is there persistent pain in the upper abdomen?
YES See *Abdominal pain*

NO

Self care advice
• If this list cannot resolve the problem please call a doctor/NHS Direct.

H45198

Further reading

Banks, Ian *Ask Dr Ian about Sex* (The Blackstaff Press, Belfast, 1999)

Banks, Ian *Get Fit With Brittas* (BBC, 1998)

Banks, Ian *The Baby Manual* (Haynes Publishing, 2003)

Banks, Ian *The NHS Direct Healthcare Guide* (Radcliffe Press, 2000)

Banks, Ian *The Sex Manual* (Haynes Publishing, 2004)

Devlin, David and Webber, Christine *The Big O* (Hodder, 1995)

Diamond, John C *Because Cowards get Cancer too* (Vermilion, London, 1999)

Egger, Garry *Trim For Life: 201 tips for effective weight control* (Allen & Unwin, St Leonards, Australia, 1997)

Finegan, Wesley C *Trust Me I'm a Cancer Patient* (Radcliffe Medical Press, 2004)

Goleman, Daniel *Emotional Intelligence: Why it can matter more than 10* (Bloomsbury, London, 1996)

Hayman, Suzie *Making the Honeymoon Last* (Hodder & Stoughton, 2000)

Martin, Paul *The Sickening Mind: Brain, Behaviour, Immunity and Disease* (Flamingo, London, 1997)

O'Donovan, Peter with Waters Jo *Preserving Your Womb* (Bladon Medical Publishing, 2004)

Ornish, Dean *Love and Survival: The Scientific Basis for the Healing Power of Intimacy* (HarperCollins, New York, 1998)

Stoppard, Miriam *New Pregnancy and Birth Book* (Dorling Kindersley, 2001)

Warburton, Diana *A-Z of Aphrodisia* (HarperCollins, London, 1995)

Glossary of terms

3D conformal radiotherapy
External beam radiotherapy that uses a computer generated three-dimensional image of the organ and special shielding to aim the X ray beam accurately at the cancer

A

Abdomen, abdominal
A part of the body which includes the stomach, intestines and other digestive organs

Abnormal
Not normal – possibly cancerous

Active monitoring
The postponement of treatment whilst regularly monitoring a cancer. Treatment may never be needed. Treatment can have a greater impact on quality of life than the cancer itself. The best action can be to monitor the cancer and commence treatment if the situation changes. This can be many years after the first diagnosis. Also called watchful waiting, active surveillance, conservative management, and expectant management

Active surveillance
See Active monitoring

Acupuncture
A complementary therapy and system of healing practised in eastern countries for thousands of years. Fine needles are inserted into 'energy points' just below the skin. Used to treat a wide range of illnesses.

Adenoma – or polyp
A benign (non-cancerous) tumour having a glandular origin and structure. Can turn cancerous

Adenocarcinoma
A malignant tumour which develops from glandular tissue. The vast majority of cancers are adenocarcinomas. The rest are a variety of much rarer types

Adjuvant therapy
A treatment given as well as the main treatment to help reduce the risk of the cancer returning. Chemotherapy, radiotherapy or hormone therapy can all be used as adjuvant therapies

Aggressive
Describes a cancer that is likely to develop and spread quickly

Androgens
Male sex hormones. See testosterone

Anaemia
Any condition in which the blood is deficient in red blood cells or haemoglobin

Anaesthesia, anaesthetics
Drugs or gases given before and during surgery so that the patient will not feel pain. The patient may be awake (local anaesthetic) or asleep (general anaesthetic)

Anti-emetic
A medicine (either tablets, an injection or a drip) that can help you feel less sick

Antioxidant
An antioxidant is a substance that may protect from the damaging effects of free radicals. A diet rich in antioxidants is protective against many forms of cancer and ill health. Antioxidants include zinc and lycopene

Axilla
The armpit

B

Benign
A swelling or growth that is not cancerous, does not spread, and is usually not life-threatening

Bereavement
The period of grief which follows the death of a loved one

Biological therapy
Treatment with substances that encourage the body's natural defence system – the immune system – to attack cancer cells. Also known as immunotherapy

Biopsy
One of the main tests used to diagnose cancer. A piece of body tissue is removed from the area where there might be cancer, and the cells are examined under a microscope. This is one of the tests used to decide whether or not a person has cancer, and what type of cancer it is

Bladder
A muscular sac that is connected to the kidneys above. It holds urine which passes out of the bladder and the body through a tube called the urethra

Blood cells
Cells that make up the blood. There are three main types – red blood cells (which carry oxygen around the body), white blood cells (which fight invading germs), and platelets (which help the blood to clot)

Blood count
This shows the number of blood cells in the bloodstream

Bone marrow
The soft and spongy centre of the bone that makes blood cells

Bone scan
A scan which looks for damage to bone

Brachytherapy
The insertion of radioactive seeds, or pellets, into a tumour to destroy cancer cells. It is used as treatment for a number of different cancers. The seeds give a dose of radiation directly into the affected area.

Bronchoscopy
A test using a flexible telescope to examine the inside of the lung

C

Cancerous
A term used to describe a tumour which has the ability to spread to nearby organs and tissues, and to other areas of the body

Carcinoma
A type of cancer which begins in the lining or covering of an organ

Catheter
A tube inserted into the bladder through the urethra to assist the flow of urine

Cell
The tiny building blocks which make up all living tissue. Cells can reproduce when needed. They have different structures in different parts of the body

Chemotherapy
Treatment with drugs to kill or slow the growth of cancer cells

Clavicle
The collarbone

Clear margin
An area of normal tissue that surrounds cancerous tissue

Clinician
Hospital doctor

Colectomy
Surgery to remove part of or all of the colon

Colic
A severe spasmodic abdominal pain

Colon
Part of the bowel

Colonoscopy
Visual examination of the inner surface of the colon by means of a flexible tube called a colonoscope

Colorectum, colorectal
Part of the bowel referring to the large intestine

Colostomy
Surgery to attach the colon to the stoma, after the rectum is removed

Complementary therapies
A wide variety of therapies which work alongside conventional medical treatment and focus on improving a person's wellbeing, psychologically as well as physically

Complete androgen blockade (CAB)
A form of hormone therapy where tablets and injections are taken in combination. Another name for MAB

Consultant
Most senior doctor

Conservative management
See Active monitoring

Cryotherapy
Also called cryoablation. The use of freezing to destroy cancer cells. A number of probes are inserted into the organ and liquid nitrogen is used to freeze and destroy the cancer cells

CT scan
A computed tomography (CT) scan produces a cross-section image of the head and body which is then analysed by a computer

Cystitis
Inflammation of the bladder that causes a burning sensation when peeing

D

Diagnosis
Identifying a disease in a person's body, or deciding what is wrong with them

E

Endoscopy
Looking inside the body through a small fibre-optic tube

Erythrocytes
Red blood cells which carry oxygen from the lungs to cells in all parts of the body and carbon dioxide back from the cells to the lungs

Expectant management
See Active monitoring

External beam radiotherapy (EBRT)
A course of high dose X-ray treatment where a beam of radioactive particles is aimed at a cancer from outside the body in order to destroy it

F

Faeces
Poo, number 2, otherwise known as bowel motions. Also see Stool

Fine Needle Aspiration (FNA)
A type of biopsy where a very thin needle is put into a tumour and a sample of fluid and cells is sucked out. The cells are looked at under a microscope to see if they are cancerous

Flatus
Wind or a fart

Fraction
A single radiotherapy treatment

Free radicals
A special type of molecule. They can be destructive in the body. Pollution, radiation and other environmental factors can introduce more into the body. Free radicals are believed to be involved in conditions such as cancer, arthritis, high blood pressure and diabetes. Anti oxidants in the diet may provide some protection against the effects of free radicals

Frequency
The frequent need to pass urine, often just small amounts

G

Genes
The coding material in all cells which affects what they are like and how they behave

Gleason score
Scale that shows how aggressive a cancer is by analysing the type of cells present in a sample. It is important to know this because the score affects the treatment choices. The scale goes from 2-10, with 2-6 being termed non-aggressive, 7 moderately aggressive and 8-10 aggressive

Guidelines, guidance
Recommended course of action for a particular illness or stage of an illness that is agreed by a team of experts

H

Haemorrhoids
Piles

Hemicolectomy
Removal of half of the colon

Hesitancy
The need to wait a moment or two before the flow of urine starts, even when the bladder is full

Hickman line
A special tube put in under anaesthetic through the chest wall into a large vein, so that chemotherapy drugs can go directly into the bloodstream

High-dose chemotherapy
Using high doses of anti-cancer drugs to kill cancer cells

Hormones
Natural chemicals in the body which affect the way organs and tissues work

Hormone receptor tests
Laboratory tests which tell if a cancer depends on hormones for growth

Hormone replacement therapy (HRT)
A treatment used to reduce the effects of the menopause by giving doses of female sex hormones as pills or patches. Some forms of HRT are associated with an increased risk of breast cancer

Hospice
Specialised units providing palliative care, including symptom control and terminal care, at the final stages of illness

Hot flushes
Commonly experienced by women going through the menopause. They vary in severity and duration. One of the conditions Intended to be alleviated by HRT

I

Ileostomy
Removal of colon and rectum, attachment of the bottom of the small intestine to the stoma

Immune system
The body's natural defence system against infection or disease

Immunotherapy
Treatment with substances that encourage the body's natural defence system – the immune system – to attack cancer cells. Also known as biological therapy

Implant
Something put into the body for a period of time, sometimes permanently

Inoperable
Refers to a cancer that cannot be removed by surgery

Incontinence
Involuntary loss of urine at inconvenient moments. This may be slight, when a pad has to be used to protect against a few drops that leak out occasionally. It may be more severe and require a catheter – a tube passed into the bladder –and attached to a leg bag, to make sure the urine drains safely and discreetly

Infusion
Introduction of fluid and/or drugs into an artery or vein

In situ
The earliest stage of cancer, when it has not spread to any other organ or area of the body

Intra-muscular
Injection into a muscle

Intravenous (IV)
Injection into a vein

Invasive
A cancer which spreads to nearby tissue

L

Latent period
Interval between the beginning of a disease and the time that the patient gets symptoms or realises there is something wrong.

Laxative
Over-the-counter medicine to soften constipated stools

Lead-time bias
If someone is screened for a disease, and the disease is found sooner than it would have been if you waited for symptoms to appear, the amount of time by which diagnosis moves forwards is the lead-time. As the point of diagnosis is then advanced in time, survival, as measured from diagnosis, is automatically lengthened, even if total length of life is not

Leukaemia
Cancer of the white blood cells

Leukocytes
White blood cells that defend the body against infections and other diseases

Lobe, lobule
Part of an organ or gland in the body

Libido
Sex drive or desire

Lump
A lump that can be felt under the skin may be a sign of cancer, but most are not cancerous

Locally advanced cancer
A locally advanced cancer is one that is no longer confined to the organ in which it arose, but has not gone far. It is not found in bone, or in local lymph nodes

Lumpectomy
Surgically removing a lump and a small amount of tissue around it

Lycopene
A powerful antioxidant found in tomatoes, which may reduce the chance of some cancers developing. Processed tomatoes, especially in tomato sauce, are especially rich in it. It is also found in other red fruits and vegetables, for example strawberries

Lymphatic system
The system that removes waste from body tissues, filters lymphatic fluid and produces cells that fight infection

Lymph nodes
Small bean-shaped organs, sometimes called lymph glands, which are part of the lymphatic system

Lymphocyte
A type of white blood cell which protects against infection

Lymphoedema
Swelling in the arms or legs that is caused when the lymph vessels are blocked or damaged. This can be caused by treatments for cancer or by the cancer itself

Lymphoma
A cancer of the lymph glands or lymphatic system

M

Malignant
Capable of invading, spreading and destroying tissue

Maximal androgen blockade (MAB)
Form of hormone therapy where tablets and injections are taken in combination. Another name for CAB

Medical oncologist
Medical doctor specialising in the treatment of cancer

Meditation
A method of relaxation

Metastasis, metastasise, metastatic
The spread of cancer cells from one part of the body to another through the bloodstream or lymphatic system. Cells that have metastasised are like those in the original tumour

Micro-calcifications
Tiny deposits of calcium that may show that cancer is present

Monitoring
Regularly checking up to see how a patient is doing or responding to treatment

MRI scan
A magnetic resonance imaging (MRI) scan uses magnets to produce pictures, which are then analysed by a computer

N

Nausea
Feeling sick

Neoplasm
Another word for cancer. From the Latin for "new growth" neoplasia – neo = new; plasia = growth

Nocturia
The need to get up to urinate during the night

Node
Part of the lymphatic system, which is the body's natural defence against infection. Lymph nodes are small masses of tissue found in clusters which purify the lymph fluid and form lymphocytes (white blood cells)

Nutrition
A healthy diet and the correct intake of vitamins and minerals

O

Oedema
A build-up of fluid in part of the body

Oesophagus, oesophageal
A tube from the mouth to the stomach

Oestrogen
Female sex hormone

Oncology
The study and treatment of cancer

Orally
Given by mouth

Ostomist
A person who has a stoma

Osteoporosis
Bone thinning due to age, level of exercise or through hormonal change. One of the conditions intended to be alleviated by HRT

P

Palliative care
Palliative care is designed to relieve symptoms rather than cure. It can be used at any stage of an illness if there are symptoms such as pain or sickness. Palliative care may help someone to live longer and to live comfortably, even if they cannot be cured

Pancreas
An organ in the digestive system that makes insulin and some of the enzymes needed for digesting food

Pathology
Examining tissues, particularly the changes in cells and tissues resulting from disease

Perineum
The area of the body between the genitals and the anus

Peripheral blood stem cell transplant (PBSCT)
A procedure in which stem cells are removed from the patient's blood, stored and then put back into the bloodstream

Platelets
The blood cells which prevent bleeding by causing blood to clot at the site of an injury

Polyp
Mass of tissue that bulges or projects outward or upward from the surface of the bowel lining

Primary cancer
Where a cancer first started in the body

Primary care
Usually used to refer to health services provided in the community rather than in hospital (for example, general practice or district nursing)

Proctitis
Inflammation of the rectum

Prognosis
The predicted or likely outcome of what might happen in the course of a disease

Prosthesis
An artificial replacement of part of the body

R

Radiation therapy, radiotherapy
A treatment which uses high-energy X-rays to kill cancer cells or keep them from dividing and growing

Receptor test
A laboratory test used to work out if a cancer depends on a certain hormone for growth

Recurrence
The return of cancer cells and signs of cancer after they appear to have gone. Sometimes known as a relapse

Reflexology
A complementary therapy which involves massaging areas of the feet

Regression
When a cancer has shrunk or disappeared

Remission
A person is said to be 'in remission' when their cancer stops growing or shows no symptoms

Rectum
The final part of the digestive system before the anus

Risk factor
An aspect of personal behaviour or lifestyle, or an environmental exposure or inherited characteristic, known to be associated with a health problem, eg, smoking is a risk factor because it increases your risk of heart disease

S

Screening
The routine examination of apparently healthy people, to identify those with a particular disease at an early stage, before anyone could be aware of it through symptoms

Secondaries, secondary cancer
New tumours, or metastases, which are formed because cancer cells from the original tumour have been carried to other parts of the body

Sentinel lymph node
The first lymph nodes that cancer cells spread to after leaving the area of the primary tumour

Shiatsu
A type of gentle massage which works on the energy flow around the body and can be helpful for stress-related conditions

Sigmoid
Last bit of the colon, above the rectum

Stem cell
The immature cells in blood and bone marrow from which all mature blood cells develop

Stoma
An artificial opening between an organ and the skin surface, that is formed by surgery. For example, a colostomy is an opening to the colon

Stool
Discharge of the bowels, the digestive waste matter discharged at one movement of the bowels; also called faeces

Subcutaneous
Given by injection under the skin

Surgery
An operation

Syringe drivers
A way of giving painkilling or chemotherapy drugs under the skin which means that patients do not need to have regular injections

Systemic therapy
Using treatments that affect the whole body

T

Terminal care
Caring for a person in the last days or weeks before they die, making sure they are free of pain and as comfortable as possible

Testosterone
Male sex hormone, or androgen

Therapy
Treatment

Thoracic
Referring to the chest area

Tissue
A group of cells

Tumour
A group of abnormal cells which keep on growing, crowding out normal cells

Tumour markers
Substances produced by some cancers that can be traced in the blood

U

Ultrasound scan
A scan which uses sound waves to build up an image of the internal organs

Urethra
The tube that carries urine from the bladder to the outside of the body

Urgency
The strong need to urinate, almost immediately

Urology
Surgical speciality dealing with the urinary tract

W

Watchful waiting
See Active monitoring

X

X-ray
A high-energy form of radiation. It is used in low doses to diagnose diseases and in high doses to treat cancer

Y

Yoga
A combination of relaxation, breathing techniques and exercise to help deal with stress and improve circulation and movement of the joints

Credits

Editor	Ian Barnes
Editorial director	Matthew Minter
Front cover picture	Mark Stevens
Page build	James Robertson
Production control	Kevin Heals
Technical illustrations	Roger Healing and Mark Stevens

A

Abdominal pain – REF•6, REF•20
Acknowledgements – 0•4
Acute otitis media – 5•3
AIDS – 4•11
Air intake (breathing) – 3•1 *et seq*
Anaemia – 4•1
Angina (angina pectoris) – 4•2
Artificial insemination – 6•12
Assisted delivery – 6•23
Asthma – 3•1
Athlete's foot – 2•1
Atrial fibrillation – 4•4

B

Backache – REF•7
Bladder cancer – 7•1
Bloke's guide to pregnancy – 6•14
Bodywork and chassis (skin and bones) – 2•1 *et seq*
Boils – 2•2
Bowel cancer – 2•14, 7•2
Breast cancer – 2•14, 7•5
Breast changes – REF•9
Breast feeding – 6•23
Breathing – 3•1 *et seq*
Breathing difficulty – REF•10
Breathlessness – 3•3
Broken bones – 1•3
Broken spine – 1•3
Bronchitis – 3•4
Burns – 1•3

C

Caesarean section – 6•23
Cancer – 2•14, 2•15, 7•1 *et seq*
Cardio-Pulmonary Resuscitation (Kiss of Life) – 1•2
Cervical cancer – 7•8
Chemotherapy – 7•5
Chest pain – REF•11
Chlamydia – 6•9

Choking – 1•3
Colostomy bag – 7•5
Condoms – 6•5
Conjunctivitis – 5•5
Constipation – 4•5
Contacts – REF•1 *et seq*
Contraception – 6•5
Corns – 2•3
Coughing – REF•12
Crabs – 2•9
Cramp – 2•4
Cystitis – 4•6

D

Dandruff – 2•4
Depression – REF•14
Diabetes (mellitus) – 4•7
Diarrhoea – REF•15
Digestion, blood & urogenital – 4•1 *et seq*
Dislocated joints – 1•3
Duodenal ulcers – 4•14
Dysmenorrhoea – 6•2

E

Ear wax – 5•1
Ectopic pregnancy – 6•18
Emergency contraception – 6•8
Endometriosis – 6•4
Eye injury – 1•4

F

Family runabout – 6•1 *et seq*
Fault finding – REF•6 *et seq*
Fever – REF•16
Fibroids – 6•4
First aid – 1•1
Forceps & Ventouse cup – 6•23
Fuel & exhaust (digestion, blood & urogenital) – 4•1 *et seq*
Further reading – REF•26

G

Gastric ulcers – 4•14
Genital herpes – 6•10
Genital warts – 6•10
German measles (Rubella) – 2•5
Glaucoma – 5•5
Glossary of terms – REF•27 *et seq*
Gonorrhoea – 6•11

H

Haemorrhoids – 4•15
Hair loss – 2•5
Headaches – REF•17
Hearing loss – 5•1
Heart attacks – 1•4, 4•8
Heartburn – 4•10
Heavy bleeding – 1•4
Hepatitis B – 6•9
Herpes – 6•10
High blood pressure (hypertension) – 4•10
HIV & AIDS – 4•11
Home Medicine Chest – 0•5
Hormone implant – 6•8
Hormone injection – 6•8
Hormone replacement therapy – 2•6
How to get the best from your GP – 0•5
Hypertension – 4•10

I

ICE (sound and vision) – 5•1 *et seq*
Indigestion and heartburn – 4•10
Infertility and artificial insemination – 6•12
Internet – REF•1
Intrauterine contraceptive device (IUD) – 6•5
Intrauterine contraceptive system (IUS) – 6•5
Irregular periods – REF•18
Itchy anus (pruritus) – 2•8

Preserving Our Motoring Heritage

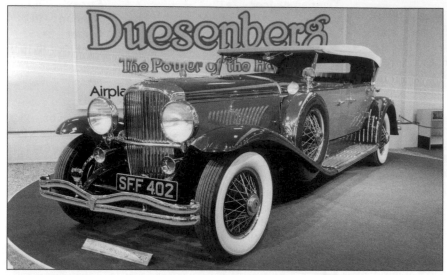

> <
> *The Model J Duesenberg Derham Tourster. Only eight of these magnificent cars were ever built – this is the only example to be found outside the United States of America*

Almost every car you've ever loved, loathed or desired is gathered under one roof at the Haynes Motor Museum. Over 300 immaculately presented cars and motorbikes represent every aspect of our motoring heritage, from elegant reminders of bygone days, such as the superb Model J Duesenberg to curiosities like the bug-eyed BMW Isetta. There are also many old friends and flames. Perhaps you remember the 1959 Ford Popular that you did your courting in? The magnificent 'Red Collection' is a spectacle of classic sports cars including AC, Alfa Romeo, Austin Healey, Ferrari, Lamborghini, Maserati, MG, Riley, Porsche and Triumph.

A Perfect Day Out

Each and every vehicle at the Haynes Motor Museum has played its part in the history and culture of Motoring. Today, they make a wonderful spectacle and a great day out for all the family. Bring the kids, bring Mum and Dad, but above all bring your camera to capture those golden memories for ever. You will also find an impressive array of motoring memorabilia, a comfortable 70 seat video cinema and one of the most extensive transport book shops in Britain. The Pit Stop Cafe serves everything from a cup of tea to wholesome, home-made meals or, if you prefer, you can enjoy the large picnic area nestled in the beautiful rural surroundings of Somerset.

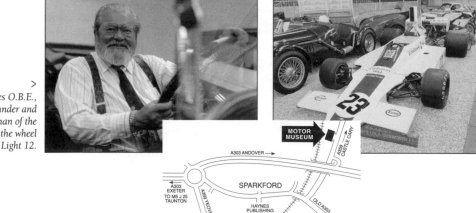

John Haynes O.B.E., Founder and Chairman of the museum at the wheel of a Haynes Light 12. >

< *Graham Hill's Lola Cosworth Formula 1 car next to a 1934 Riley Sports.*

The Museum is situated on the A359 Yeovil to Frome road at Sparkford, just off the A303 in Somerset. It is about 40 miles south of Bristol, and 25 minutes drive from the M5 intersection at Taunton.
Open 9.30am - 5.30pm (10.00am - 4.00pm Winter) 7 days a week, *except Christmas Day, Boxing Day and New Years Day*
Special rates available for schools, coach parties and outings Charitable Trust No. 292048